From Hormone Hell To Hormone Well

Discover Human-Identical Hormones as a Safe and
Effective Treatment for PMS, Perimenopause, Menopause or
Hysterectomy

by

C.W. Randolph, Jr., M.D.
and Genie James, M.M.Sc.

First Edition

The Natural Hormone Institute of America, Inc.
Jacksonville Beach, Florida

Also by C.W. Randolph, Jr., M.D.

Natural Hormone Balance

From Hormone Hell To Hormone Well
by C.W. Randolph, Jr., M.D. and Genie James, M.M.Sc.

This book contains general information and is not intended to be a used as a substitute for the professional medical advice of a qualified physician concerning an individual's specific healthcare needs. You are advised and encouraged to consult your healthcare professional with regards to all matters relating to your health.

Published by The Natural Hormone Institute of America, Inc.
1891 Beach Boulevard, Suite 100
Jacksonville Beach, Florida 32250 U.S.A.
www.safesthormones.com
Phone: 866-628-6337

ISBN 0-9754270-0-8
First Edition

Cover Design by Latocki Team Creative, LLC
Book Design by John Kaszuba

Printed in the United States of America by Vaughan Printing,Inc

Dedication

This book is dedicated to John R. Lee, M.D., one of our medical community's most respected pioneers and revered champions of women's health. Even after Dr. Lee's death, I continue to be in awe of how he committed his life's work to increasing awareness regarding the safety and efficacy of bio-identical/human-identical hormone replacement as an alternative to synthetic hormone replacement therapy. His personal effort to spend several decades of his life circling the globe to challenge traditional medical teachings and "get the word out" is unprecedented.

Today, I know that Dr. Lee's cause will continue. May he rest in peace knowing that those many physicians who he mentored, including myself, will forever channel our energies and raise our voices to ensure that his mission will not die.

Finally, I want to also dedicate this book to all women currently living in their own personal "hormone hell." May the information and knowledge shared throughout these pages create for you a passage to "hormone wellness."

God bless,

C. W. Randolph, Jr., M. D.

Acknowledgements

There are many people who I want to thank for their participation in moving this book from an idea in my mind to a work of art in print. First and foremost, I want to thank God for giving me the ability, knowledge, and talent to become a physician and healer. I acknowledge that each day I serve women (and men) through my medical practice. I am also privileged to be in a profession where I am able to actively serve as an instructor of my Creator.

Secondly, I would like to thank my co-author Genie James for her spiritual presence on every page of this book. I am grateful for her knowledge, drive, research, and ability to move fluidly from medical terminology to patient testimonies. I know that Genie's input helped us craft this book with language and tone that should have meaning for both healthcare professionals and laypersons.

While I dedicated this book to John R. Lee, M.D., it is important for me to take this opportunity once again to underscore the seminal role he played in opening my mind and eyes to the clinical efficacy and safety of human-identical hormones as an alternative to synthetic hormone replacement. In addition, I am deeply indebted to many of my medical colleagues who have served as pioneers in the field of human-identical replacement therapy.

Specifically, I want to thank Dr. David Zava for his research on saliva testing and the relationship between hormone replacement and breast cancer; Dr. Helene Leonetti for her daring research on the clinical benefits of human-identical progesterone cream; Dr. Joel Hargrove for catalyzing ground-breaking research while serving as a clinical professor for the Department of Obstetrics and Gynecology for Vanderbilt University's School of Medicine; and, Dr. Robert Gottesman for his work including his publishing of *The Progesterone Saga*. I want to gratefulley acknowledge Dr. Carl Burak for first introducing me to Dr. John Lee's work. Also, I want to thank his wife and my friend Ronnie Burak for her ever encouraging words cheering me through the writing of this book.

Finally, I want to acknowledge Virginia Hopkins for her pivotal role in working with Dr. John R. Lee to co-author three books that have helped set the stage for the current revolution supporting the use of human-identical hormone therapies; e.g. *What Your Doctor May Not Tell You About Premenopause, What Your Doctor May Not Tell You About Menopause*, and *What Your Doctor May Not Tell You About Breast Cancer*.

When I determined to put my work, research and thoughts on paper for mass consumption, I have to admit that I had no idea how to print and publish a book. The fact that this book is now a reality is a result of a lot of work by a very talented and committed "virtual" team of individuals. I want to thank John Kaszuba for his assistance with both research and the formatting of text. I also want to recognize Amy Jo Robertson for her assistance and valuable skills in working with Ms. James to make sure this would be a book every woman could easily read and, as a result, translate from an individual healthcare consumer's point of view whether or not human-identical hormone therapies had the potential to improve their health or quality of life.

In the last stages of production, both Ms. James and I were deeply grateful when my daughter, Dänika Randolph, offered to roll up her sleeves and use her training from the publishing realm to serve as our final editorial advisor. I also want to acknowledge Sharon Miller of Vaughan Printing, Inc. and Bruce Butler of the Greenleaf Book Group, LLC. Both Ms. Miller and Mr. Butler played a key role in shepherding Ms. James and me through a quagmire of unfamiliarity related to what it takes to self-publish and make a book like this readily available to the consumer.

Special thanks is due to Nanette Noffsinger for her can-do approach to developing and launching our media and public relations strategy. Ms. Noffsinger's style, skills, vision, and perspective added a delightful touch of grace to this endeavor. Her role extended even to training me on how best to feel at ease in front of a camera or large audience. I learned from Ms. Noffsinger that even a *salty old dog* can learn new tricks! My gratitude for her contribution is boundless.

Before I close, I want to thank the talented and gifted team of healthcare professionals and office staff that I am privileged to work with every day in my Jacksonville medical practice. I continue to learn from and be in awe of their day-to-day willingness to, first, listen to our patients' concerns and, then, treat each individual with heartfelt compassion and respect.

Finally, I want to acknowledge my patients. This book would have no purpose or meaning without them, their clinical results, and their personal testimonies. My hope is that, by sharing the stories of my patients who have benefited from the treatment regimens described in this text, I can help increase awareness, understanding, and utilization of human-identical hormone therapies.

CONTENTS

CONTENTS

CONTENTS

CONTENTS

CONTENTS

Introduction

Honoring the Mystery of Women

As a man, I am deeply aware that no matter how hard I strive I will never be able completely to grasp how women think, feel, respond and relate. When I was younger, I was very much in awe of women and thought they were sort of like exquisite cats: mostly mysterious and more than sometimes temperamental. For many years the female sex confounded me, even though I grew up as the only boy in a family with three sisters. I had my share of girlfriends along the way and got involved to some extent, but to protect myself from the mercurial power of the feminine, I also kept my distance.

Then, my world changed. I witnessed the birth of my daughter, Dänika. Watching my girl-child come out of her mother's womb brought me to my knees. I had no words with which to honor my wife for the strength and courage she exhibited throughout gestation, as well as during labor and delivery. I had no prior experience to prepare me for the depth of my feelings for this new life, this little being who seemed to trust me to know what she needed and how to take care of her. I felt inexplicably humbled.

Somewhere within me, walls tumbled down. From that point forward, my perspective regarding women moved into new dimensions of esteem, wonder, and respect. It became of paramount importance to me to learn more about how women thought, felt, lived, nurtured, and healed. I suddenly felt constrained by the neat and analytical nature of my professional career as a licensed pharmacist. I found myself moving into new realms of research and study as I strove to unlock the mystery of the feminine psyche while also searching for knowledge to explain the wisdom and power women hold in their bodies. Even more than that, I began to ask myself if I might someday serve women with my gifts and talents.

Today, more than twenty-five years later, I am a successful Board Certified Obstetrician and Gynecologist (OB/GYN). Since inception, my practice has been dedicated to women's health and a more natural medicine approach to wholeness and healing. For many years, I took great joy in delivering healthy, beautiful babies. Over time, however, I found that my greatest gifts as a healer manifested when I worked with my patients to address their health issues associated with aging. Consequently, in 1998, I made the decision to devote the main thrust of my energies towards gynecology and a more natural approach to hormone balance therapies.

Challenging the Medical System

I, along with every other physician who graduated from medical school in the last several decades, was trained to believe that synthetic hormone replacement therapy (HRT) provided a number of health benefits for women suffering from the symptoms of hormonal changes. The touted benefits of HRT included relief of vasomotor symptoms (hot flashes), reversal of vaginal atrophy (thinning and drying of the vaginal tissues), and prevention of osteoporosis (progressive loss of bone mass). Medical schools also taught that a complete hysterectomy (removal of the uterus, tubes and ovaries) was the recommended treatment option for women with dysfunctional bleeding, fibroid tumors or endometriosis with

3

chronic pelvic pain. For years, leading women's health experts contended that - for a woman who has had all the children she wants or who is past childbearing age - the ovaries were just inert fibrous tissue masses that served no function for the aging female body. Today, I am convinced, and have the clinical evidence to prove, that the training we physicians received from our respective medical schools was wrong.

When I opened my practice, I initially adhered to my medical school training and regularly prescribed synthetic HRT, such as the pharmaceutical brands Premarin, Provera, and Prempro, for my patients who had undergone a hysterectomy or who were suffering from menopausal symptoms. When asked about side effects, including weight gain, I repeated what I had been taught and indicated that there was no clinical evidence to support these concerns. Nevertheless, it took only a couple of years for me to seriously doubt my training and to begin to treat my patients with an alternative: human-identical hormonal therapies.

What triggered my concerns, you might ask? Very simply, I listened to my patients and paid attention to their responses and reactions to synthetic HRT. Many of the women for whom I had prescribed synthetic HRT did gain a great deal of weight. I could not attribute their weight gain to changes in eating habits or lifestyle activities; the only thing that had changed for them was the introduction of synthetic estrogen into their systems. In addition to their concerns about weight gain, these same patients frequently came in with new complaints including bloating, decreased libido, depression, poor quality of sleep, and "just not feeling right."

What I heard and observed confused me. I began to ask myself: "If what I had been taught about HRT and weight gain could be wrong, what other aspects of my training regarding synthetic hormone replacement might be erroneous?" I was determined to take a deeper look. First, I tested to see if my patients' responses validated what was then the accepted medical theory that HRT would help prevent osteoporosis. It didn't. When I tested the bone mineral density of my patients who had been on HRT, I found that instead of evidencing an increase in bone density, many had borderline or true osteoporosis. My confusion began to turn to real concern. I began to ask: "Is HRT helping or hurting my patients?"

Finally, I became highly concerned about the potential correlation between synthetic HRT and my patients' breast health. I found that women I put on synthetic HRT were likely to return six months to a year later with breast lumps and even worse, years later some would return to be diagnosed with breast cancer. Even though the volume of patients I was personally tracking did not equate to a statistically sound research database, I saw enough to make me question whether the synthetic HRT I was prescribing for my patients was causing an estrogen dominance that contributed to excessive breast cell proliferation. From that point on, my concerns regarding the potentially negative health concerns associated with synthetic HRT transmuted from confusion and concern to a mixture of fear and anger. I asked myself: "Could it be that synthetic hormones actually have a carcinogenic effect?" and, "If I believe that HRT is harmful, then what do I do now?"

All of these questions began to come to a head for me in the early 1990's, a decade before the medical establishment began to question the safety and efficacy of synthetic hormone therapies. Today there is a groundswell of paranoia regarding HRT as a choice for treating menopausal symptoms, as well as for the prevention of some postmenopausal conditions.

These much-publicized concerns are primarily derived from the findings of the National Institutes of Health (NIH) sponsored Women's Health Initiative (WHI) study released in 2002. The WHI study was initiated with the original purpose of scientifically validating the benefits of combination HRT for menopausal symptoms as well as the prevention of some postmenopausal conditions, such as osteoporosis. While the study was initially intended to last eight years, it was halted after only five years because the findings indicated that the women in the study who were taking the combination HRT actually evidenced an increased risk of heart disease, breast cancer, stroke and blood clots. More than ten years after I was dubbed "a maverick" for taking my patients off synthetic hormones, the WHI study validated my concerns and reported that synthetic HRT actually poses more health risks to women than benefits.

Many now say that I was ahead of my time because I began to turn away from prescribing synthetic hormones before the controversy regarding HRT officially erupted. Some of my physician peers have even recanted their earlier declarations of my being too radical in my thinking and too holistic in my approaches to be practicing medicine. Now these same physicians celebrate me as a pioneer and ask me to teach them how to treat their own patients with human-identical hormone therapies.

I honestly don't think of myself as any kind of medical hero; I simply do my best to take care of my patients. When I first observed the negative effects of HRT, I knew that I had to challenge conventional medical thinking. I determined that if the treatment-of-choice I had been taught in medical school was harmful instead of helpful then I would find another answer. I drew on my background as a pharmacist and began to search for alternatives.

Searching for Answers

When I first began to challenge conventional medical thinking regarding synthetic HRT I thought that I was embarking on a very lonely path; however, as I began to research the medical literature, I gratefully discovered that the beginning of a medical revolution was already underway. I came across a small book entitled *Natural Progesterone: The Multiple Roles of a Remarkable Hormone* written by John R. Lee, M.D. Dr. Lee contended that excess estrogen, when unopposed or unbalanced by progesterone, could result in many undesirable side effects. I read Dr. Lee's writings and was introduced to several new clinical terms including: "estrogen dominance," "progesterone balance," and "bio-identical" hormones. I recognized that I had happened onto a "bible" of new thought that would profoundly change my life - and my medical practice - forever.

Dr. Lee's works introduced me to a new science of hormone replacement at a time (early 1990's) when the conventional medical thinking was that menopause signaled the onset of an estrogen deficiency disease that required estrogen treatment. He was one of the first to shake up conventional thought by proposing the following three questions:

1. Why does the medical community focus solely on estrogen and essentially ignore the other hormones in the female body?

2. What is the role of these other hormones produced by the ovaries; e.g. progesterone and androgens such as testosterone?

3. How does the interrelation of all these hormones change as women age?

I dove into this new field of study. The science of hormone balancing made sense to me. I already knew that, in a normally functioning pre-menopausal woman, estrogens are made from progesterone and/or from androgens within the cells of the ovaries. After menopause the amount of progesterone in the body significantly decreases and estrogen production relies on the adrenal-producing androgens, primarily body fat. I recognized that my medical school training had not adequately explored the impact of the shift in hormonal ratios. Like Dr. Lee, I began to believe that the key to safe and effective hormone therapy was rooted in coming to a new understanding of how hormonal balance changes with age. In addition, I began to suspect that the interdependence of estrogen and progesterone was a core variable impacting a woman's health and that the medical community had previously overlooked its critical significance.

I returned to my respect for the wisdom that I knew resided within the female body. I knew that each woman has a unique hormonal ratio that, when in balance, supports good health. I already understood that during a woman's lifecycle, the equilibrium of estrogen, progesterone, and testosterone shifted. I recognized that symptoms such as hot flashes, dysfunctional bleeding, weight gain, and even depression were the female body's way of signaling a system out of balance.

To treat the individual concerns of each of my patients, I needed to obtain an individualized hormonal profile. At the time, those physicians who did bother to test hormone levels usually relied on analyzing blood serum levels. I found those blood tests frequently to be unreliable, especially for progesterone. Consequently, I chose to use saliva tests to evaluate free-hormone levels within the body. The results were much more accurate. Eventually, I obtained salivary testing kits from Dr. David Zava's laboratory in Portland, Oregon, and made salivary testing a part of my standard protocol for diagnosing and treating my patients suffering from symptoms of hormone imbalance.

When I began to analyze the findings of these salivary tests, my results mirrored Dr. Lee's premise. I found that, when estrogen was the dominant hormone and progesterone was deficient, the impact on my patient was toxic. Adding more estrogen via synthetic HRT only exacerbated the problem. I was convinced that the real therapeutic opportunity to mitigate hormonal imbalance would occur as a result of increasing progesterone levels.

Identifying a Healthy Alternative: Human-Identical Hormones

It did not take long before I was completely converted to this new theory regarding hormone therapy replacement. I was convinced that the best results would be obtained by testing my patients to determine their salivary hormone levels and then individualizing their doses of needed progesterone, estrogen and/or testosterone. Yet I knew that the approach was only half the answer. What about the treatment?

As I mentioned earlier, it was my concern regarding the potentially adverse health effects of synthetic hormones that first compelled me to search for alternatives. Synthetic hormones such as Premarin, Provera, Prempro, Femhrt, Activella, Cenestin, Ogen and Menest have a chemical molecular structure that is similar, but not identical, to those produced in the human body. I became convinced that hormones with the exact same molecular structure as those produced by a woman's ovaries were required for hormone replacement therapy to be both safe and effective.

As a pharmacist, I knew that it was possible to synthesize in a lab a molecular structure that would exactly match the molecular structure of hormones manufactured in the ovaries. It was intuitively and scientifically obvious to me that the female body would better recognize and utilize these human-identical hormones, sometimes also referred to as bio-identical. There were already some "natural" hormone products on the market, most specifically several different brands of progesterone cream. Still, I had some concerns about switching to these over-the-counter alternatives.

First, I didn't see how I could individualize each patient's regimen to address their specific imbalances and needs if these formulations were premixed. Secondly, because of my comprehensive training in pharmacology, I had high standards for any lab that would be compounding formulations for my patients. How could I ensure that an over-the-counter product was manufactured in a lab that would meet the strict standards of the National Association of Compounding Pharmacists? I felt that the field of human-identical hormone production was too new for me to trust someone else to develop products that I could have confidence in to treat my patients. Consequently, I built a compounding lab and began formulating from scratch my own brand of human-identical hormone products.

Almost a decade after I began to compound my own human-identical products, I can report that there are now many compounding pharmacies that have the ability to formulate products of the same quality as long as the prescribing physician knows how to properly write the prescription. I am grateful that, today, many more physicians share my concerns regarding the inherent risks of synthetic hormone therapies. There is also increasing consumer demand for healthier options. Such respected sources as Vanderbilt University Medical Center, Harvard University's Department of Anthropology, the *American Journal of Obstetrics and Gynecology* and the *Clinical Chemistry Professional Journal* have published research that has fueled the support for human-identical hormone therapies. I would like to honor the pioneers in this field who I count as my mentors, Drs. John Lee, Helene Leonetti and David Zava. In addition, other such respected and learned physicians as Christiane Northrup, Joel Hargrove, Jeanne Drisko, and Johnathan Wright have raised their voices to educate both physicians and patients regarding the benefits of human-identical hormone therapies.

Getting the Word Out

We have made progress in getting the word out, but there is still more work to do. I decided to write this book because I still see too many women who come into my office suffering from the symptoms of hormone imbalance. The women who are most frustrated are the ones who have spent years with physicians who continued to recommend synthetic HRT (albeit in smaller dosages) or the women who were told there were no other options. When their symptoms didn't go away or even worsened, these women were advised that "they would just have to live with their discomfort until they were through menopause." Even more criminal, there are still those physicians who try to convince their patients that "it is all in your head." This must be stopped.

I can make the case for human-identical hormone therapy and I am committed to getting the word out. In 2003, I founded The Natural Hormone Institute of America. This entity was established with a mission that embraces both education and research. While I am passionately convinced about the benefits of human-identical hormone therapy, many of my peers within the medical community – as well as female consumers - still need to be educated as to their advantages. In addition, there is still need for research and clinical trials to evaluate other long term health effects and administration routes of human-identical hormone therapy, such as those related to birth control, weight gain and anti-aging.

Also, in 2003 I was fortunate enough to meet Genie James, a recognized expert in the fields of women's health, integrated models of care, community health status management, and consumer driven models for healthcare delivery. I learned that Genie had previously published two books: *Making Managed Care Work* and *Winning in the Women's Healthcare Marketplace.* More importantly, Genie and I discovered that we both have a passion for natural medicine and women's health concerns. I chose to partner with Genie to write this book so that, together, we could share a compilation of clinical data, medical information, and case studies to support this powerful revolution. We have attempted to use terms that would be credible to a physician, but also easy for a layperson to grasp.

Chapter 1, "What's Going On In There?" opens the book by explaining the anatomy of the female body as it relates to hormone production. It then describes the bio-chemical purpose of hormones and what happens when they are out of balance and their natural function is impaired.

Chapter 2, "Introducing A Circle of Women...And Men," translates the science of hormone replacement into day-to-day life. We use real-life case studies to illustrate for the reader the many health concerns associated with hormone imbalance.

Chapter 3, "Synthetic Hormone Replacement Therapy (HRT): A Pharmaceutical 'Dr. Jekyll and Mr. Hyde,'" then expounds on why synthetic hormones are still so widely - and inappropriately - prescribed despite the mounting medical evidence of their toxicity.

Chapter 4, "You Do Have a Choice," introduces the reader to the clinical advantages and potential benefits of human-identical hormone therapies.

Chapter 5, "Personalized Medicine: One Size Does Not Fit All," speaks to the fact that each female patient is an individual and that there are no "cookie-cutter solutions" for optimizing each woman's unique hormonal equilibrium. The advantages of less well-recognized but highly valuable clinical tools, such as salivary and urinary testing, are discussed in detail.

Chapter 6, "Progesterone: The 'Feel Good' Hormone" is seminal to both the mission of this book to provide a safe and effective alternative to synthetic hormone therapies and my commitment as a physician to educate both the medical community and the female consumer as to the advantages and benefit of human-identical hormone replacement. In this chapter, we highlight the fact that the traditional medical approach has been to treat menopausal symptoms with estrogen therapy. We then go on to share scientific and clinical evidence to support our medical theory that most symptoms of hormone imbalance are the result of estrogen dominance, not estrogen deficiency.

Our premise is that, when estrogen is unopposed by progesterone, it will wreak havoc in the body and can actually have a cancer-promoting effect at the cellular level. In contrast, when human-identical progesterone is introduced into the system of a woman suffering from the symptoms of hormone imbalance, it is shown to have many life-changing health benefits. Chapter 6 is so important because it opens the reader's mind to a new way of thinking: human-identical progesterone as the cornerstone of almost every hormone replacement regimen.

Still, hormone balance requires the synergy of multiple hormones; progesterone does not work alone in the body. In Chapter 7, "Your Sex Hormones in Balance: A Healthy Ménage à Trois," we move on to describe the shifting dynamics, critical roles and interacting functions of all the body's sex hormones; e.g. estrogen, progesterone and testosterone.

Because of the number of baby-boomer women entering menopause and considering surgical alternatives, many readers will probably turn immediately to Chapter

8, "Hysterectomy Hysteria." In this chapter we do discuss the medical reasons why it is appropriate for women to have a hysterectomy and how human-identical hormone therapy can help restore optimum health for women who are surgically plunged into menopause. We also address the fact that, for many women, there may be viable alternatives to a complete surgical removal of all female organs. For those women considering the pros and cons of a hysterectomy, Chapter 8 outlines these options and choices in detail.

Chapter 9, "Adrenal Exhaustion: Stress, Fatigue, and Accelerated Aging" is most exciting in that it speaks to an issue that every baby-boomer today is interested in. In a normal lifecycle, adrenal hormones (e.g. DHEA and cortisol) decline in tandem with the aging process. The human body is a very exquisitely tuned mechanism. Under stress and when fatigued, its systems often shut down and/or malfunction causing the body to accelerate its decline in production of essential adrenal hormones. In this chapter we address the symptomatic catalysts of the aging process and describe both how a combination of lifestyle choices, mind-body exercises, and human-identical hormone therapy can work together to promote and extend the feeling and appearance of youth and vitality.

Chapter 10, "Hormone Health During The Reproductive Years" has value to the reader because hormone balance is not just an issue for women approaching "the change." The chapter looks at such pertinent issues as the relationship of hormone balance to infertility and how taking birth control pills may interfere with the body's natural hormone balance.

Chapter 11, "The Link between Hormones And Breast Cancer," is a topic of great interest to almost every woman alive today. This chapter will discuss those risk factors that cannot be impacted, such as genetics, as well as those that can, such as hormone balance and diet. In addition, this chapter will address the importance of naturally occurring or human-identical progesterone as an ongoing supplement to support breast health.

Chapter 12, "Men Have Hormones Too: Understanding Andropause" connects male hormone imbalances with symptoms of midlife. As men age, their testosterone levels decline. Symptoms most frequently associated with andropause - or male menopause - include weight gain around the middle, depression, less muscle mass and a decline in sexual performance. With the baby-boomer generation coming of age, it is no wonder pharmaceutical products like Viagra have been so popular as a band-aid approach to reinstating manhood and youth via an erection. Still, there are others issues at hand and other approaches to treating the complete man. Human-identical hormone therapy is for men too.

Chapter 13, "Human-Identical Hormone Therapy: A Medical Revolution." By sharing a vision of a new model and approach to hormone therapy, this book will empower the informed female healthcare consumer to be more aware and in charge of treatment options and decisions. Women never again have to feel like victims of the traditional medical establishment and pharmaceutical dollar machines to decide how to take care of their bodies as they age and change. While the movement to establish human-identical hormone therapies as a treatment of choice is exciting, its importance pales beside the significance of the movement for women to define and drive a new model for healthcare response and delivery.

Finally, Chapter 14 concludes this book by providing the reader with a resource listing. Because the field of human-identical hormone therapy is still regarded as "alternative medicine" by most of the traditional medical community, we feel that it is essential for the reader to know where to look for credible information and where to go for help. The compilation of names and contact information includes organizations, physicians, saliva testing facilities, compounding pharmacies, and recommended reading.

In summary, let me say that when Ms. James and I embarked on our journey to bring this book to life, our intention was to clarify the risks of using synthetic HRT, and to share evidence as to the benefit of human-identical hormone replacement. We hope that what is shared in this book fosters education and, more importantly, engenders hope.

Even though I have successfully treated thousands of women with human-identical hormones, I continue to be awed by every one of my patients. I am deeply aware that each woman's mind, body, and spirit uniquely entwines with the heart of creation. I learn from my patients, and as I treat their bodies, I honor their personal choices and celebrate their wisdom. While I am privileged to serve many women as their personal physician, I hope that, through this book and the work of The Natural Hormone Institute of America, we reach and help heal many more.

Chapter 1

What's Going On in "There?"

As you read this book, you will learn how hormonal balance is key to fostering physical, mental, and emotional health. As a physician, I too often see patients in my office whose physical and emotional concerns remained unresolved despite years of going from doctor to doctor hoping to get relief. These women continued to suffer needlessly because their underlying issue of hormone imbalance was not recognized or addressed. It does not have to be that way.

While our culture is seemingly obsessed with a woman's sexual organs, little awareness is given to the anatomy, physiology, and biochemistry of a woman's body. I remember watching the movie *Fried Green Tomatoes* and chuckling wholeheartedly during the scene when Evelyn Couch, the story's narrator played by Kathy Bates, attended a support group where each woman was challenged to embrace her sexuality by looking at her vagina in a mirror. She was first somewhat horrified, then, more than a little fascinated. I felt like Evelyn could easily have been one of my patients coming into my office and embarrassedly asking me questions about what was really going on "down there."

Unfortunately, as little as most women know about "down there," or their female genitalia, they know even less about what is happening "in there," e.g. the interior of their bodies. Most women who come into my office don't have a clue regarding where their hormones are produced, how they are distributed or what they do to promote health at a cellular level. For those women undergoing the hormonal changes associated with menopause or hysterectomy, it is a travesty that much of the medical community and the media are so uninformed that they perpetuate misinformation about synthetic hormone replacement therapies (HRT) versus natural hormone treatment options.

Because most of the data regarding hormone replacement is so conflicted, most women today are just plain confused about hormone replacement therapy. Consequently, they become loaded with anxiety - and even shame - when they begin to experience the physical and emotional symptoms associated with hormonal shifts. Many women feel helpless and, as a result of fear and embarrassment, they attempt to shroud their symptoms in secrecy.

What women need to know is that aging and hormonal shifts do not have to mean pain, suffering, and giving up the good life. The truth is that every cycle of a woman's time here on earth will be ushered in through a natural metamorphosis that will have physical, emotional, mental, and spiritual facets of change. Throughout life, the human body is evidence of the miracle of creation and transformation. Each body houses more than fifty million cells that work to shuttle nutrients, build new cells, and dismantle old ones. Every year, the body replaces more than 98% of its total atoms. Women who are forty, fifty, or sixty years old do not have bodies that are "finished." As long as there is life, there is change. Over a lifespan, the female body will be in a constant state of renewal.

Still, as women age, a shift in hormone balance is inevitable. Most of the traditional medical community continues to think that the distress typically associated with hormone imbalance is also unavoidable. This thinking is dead wrong. In fact, the opposite is true. No matter a woman's age, hormones can be balanced the way the body originally intended and can contribute to health, vitality, and a youthful appearance.

Unfortunately, for most physicians and patients, ignorance regarding hormone imbalance and hormone therapies continues to breed fear and poor decisions. I find that as I educate my patients to better understand and anticipate the impact of their hormonal shifts, they are both comforted and excited. The feeling of comfort seems to come from knowing that they are not crazy or dying, nor are they alone. The sense of excitement appears directly related to a renewed sense of choice. I am writing this book so that this knowledge can empower more women.

Because knowledge must precede choice, this first chapter is intended to educate how the female body naturally produces and distributes hormones. It also describes just how the body's hormonal functions change over time. Finally, to give a context that can easily be identified with, this chapter offers real-life examples of women suffering from the symptoms of hormone imbalance.

Looking Inside: The Endocrine System

Understanding the endocrine system is the first step to understanding how the body produces and balances hormones. Medical and scientific studies validate that hormone balance is a constant and fundamental variable impacting a woman's health across her lifespan. The female hormones affect every cell in the body, including the brain.

The truth is that, in order for the body to work the way it is supposed to, balanced hormones are as necessary as oxygen and blood.

The endocrine system is composed of several glands that serve as the female body's operational center for regulating hormone production and distribution. I liken the endocrine system to a hand manipulating the strings of a marionette. If the hand drops one string, then the puppet would probably not be able to dance or keep up its role in the play. Similarly, if any gland within the endocrine system is not functioning properly, hormone balance will be challenged and the whole body will suffer.

To begin to understand the complexity of hormone interactions, it is important to understand the unique function of each gland, its role in hormone production, as well as its interdependent relationship within the endocrine system. In brief:

- Both the pituitary and hypothalamus glands are pivotal in regulating the flow of all hormones throughout the body, including estrogen, progesterone and testosterone. The hypothalamus also directly interacts with the neurotransmitters that regulate mood.

- The hypothalamus produces GnRH (gonadotropin-releasing hormone). The pituitary gland produces FSH (follicle-stimulating hormone) and LH (luteinizing hormone). These hormones serve to stimulate the rise of estrogen and progesterone during the monthly menstrual cycle.

- The thyroid gland is best known for its metabolic function affecting weight. The prevalence of thyroid problems increase with age. Approximately 26 percent of middle-aged women are diagnosed with hypothyroidism. In addition to weight gain, other symptoms of thyroid dysfunction include mood disturbances, low energy level, mental confusion, and sleep disturbances.

The two thumb-sized adrenal glands play a critical role in producing hormones and regulating the sympathetic nervous system. One cardinal sign of adrenal exhaustion is relentless, debilitating fatigue. Adrenal glands secrete three hormones in response to stress:

- Epinepherine is the fight-or-flight hormone produced when you think you are being threatened or are in danger.

- Cortisol increases appetite and energy level while taming the allergic and inflammatory responses of the immune system.

- Dehydroepiandrosterone, or DHEA, is often referred to as the 'anti-aging' hormone. It can help protect/increase bone density, keep bad cholesterol levels under control, provide a general sense of vitality and energy, aid natural sleep patterns, and improve mental acuity.

The ovaries are the female body's source of reproductive life. Within the ovaries are the follicles that store a woman's eggs, or ovum. Every month during a woman's reproductive years, the pituitary gland hormone, FSH, stimulates the follicles to come forth to release their ovum. This process is called ovulation. At puberty, a woman has approximately 400,000 follicles within her ovaries. By her thirties, however, the number of follicles remaining is closer to 25-30,000.

In addition to ovulation, the ovaries produce the female sex hormone estrogen. Estrogen is primarily responsible for the growth of female characteristics in puberty and regulating the menstrual cycle throughout the reproductive years. The term "estrogen" is really short-hand for a group of several different but related hormones that perform similar functions within the body. In adult women, three different natural estrogens predominate:

- Estrone/E1 (approximately 3-5% of circulating estrogen)

- Estradiol/E2 (approximately 10-20% of circulating estrogen)

- Estriol/E3 (approximately 60-80% of circulating estrogen)

Under normal circumstances, estrogen levels vary according to the stage of the menstrual cycle, but the amount of each type of estrogen usually fluctuates within the proportions above. (Note: while the ovaries are the primary site for production, body fat can also be a source of estrogen.) The interaction between ovarian estrogen production and the estrogen derived from human body fat will be discussed later in chapter 11.

In addition to estrogen, ovaries also produce progesterone, testosterone, and the androgenic hormones (e.g. the biochemical building blocks for testosterone and the estrogens) throughout a woman's life. During the reproductive years, progesterone maintains the uterus and prepares it for pregnancy. Progesterone also supports the brain's function of controlling mental acuity and emotional stability. At optimal levels and in balance with the other hormones, progesterone can be attributed to promoting an attitude of calmness, and also fostering healthy sleeping patterns.

> *Although testosterone is often thought of as a male hormone, it actually has a very vital function within the female body. In a biochemical sense, testosterone's role has nothing to do with making babies, but it can impact sex drive. Testosterone can also benefit the body by increasing energy levels, improving muscle tone, and maintaining vaginal wall thickness while also enhancing the vagina's ability to naturally lubricate.*

The body makes hormones from nutrients with the help of enzymes. While the metabolic pathways for hormone production can be more than a little confusing to the average person, their origin is actually quite simple. Would you believe that cholesterol is the single building block molecule from which all other sex hormones are derived? No cholesterol means no estrogen, no progesterone, and no testosterone. Because of the this organic chemistry phenomenon, it is not surprising that many women who go on extremely low-fat, low-cholesterol diets actually accelerate a hormone imbalance.

A first look at Figure 1: Steroid Family Tree (see the insert on page 30) can be daunting. The good news is that it really is not necessary for you to become a biochemistry whiz kid who can diagram hormonal pathways in order to begin to understand what is going on inside your body as it relates to hormone balance. The intricacies of your endocrine system can seem overwhelming. What is important to recognize, however, is how critical these glands are. Very simply, the hormones produced and distributed by your endocrine system are essential fuel for the finely tuned biological miracle that is your body. If your endocrine system malfunctions, symptoms will occur. These physical, mental, and/or emotional manifestations are how your body signals a hormone imbalance.

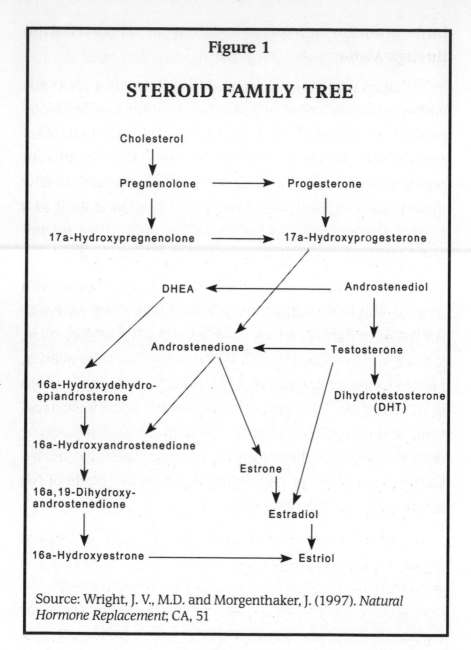

Figure 1

STEROID FAMILY TREE

Figure 1 shows the production pathway of sex hormones in the human body.

Understanding a Woman's Lifecycle: Menstruation through Menopause

Once you learn where and how hormones are made within your body, you next need to understand how hormone production and balance can change as you age. Certain issues and, therein, certain choices, will be more critical at different points of a woman's lifecycle. If the term "lifecycle" is new to you, think of it as a segment of life that lends itself to a categorization of physical symptoms, health concerns, mental attitudes, spiritual questioning, and lifestyle choices.

The first cycle, the early reproductive stage, begins with a girl's first menses and lasts until she is about thirty years old. For the most part, if periods occur on a normal 28-day cycle, it can be inferred that the body, and particularly the ovaries, are producing plenty of all the hormones. Some young women in the early reproductive stage do experience premenstrual syndrome, or PMS, although it is more likely to begin to occur once a woman is in her thirties. Bloating, anxiety, irritability, back pain, nausea, cramping and lethargy are some of the most common PMS symptoms.

As a woman enters her mid-thirties and until she is in her late forties, she can be said to be pre-menopausal. A woman in this lifecycle is in her middle reproductive years. It is during these years that the balance of hormones produced by a woman's endocrine system first begins to shift. Progesterone, the "feel good" hormone, is the first hormone to decline and drops 120 times more rapidly than estrogen. As progesterone begins to decline and estrogen becomes the dominant hormone within a woman's system, symptoms such as PMS, breast swelling, irregular periods, fluid retention, uterine fibroids, fibrocystic disease, reduced libido and migraine headaches occur.

It is important to understand that estrogen dominance does not necessarily mean that the body is producing too much estrogen; rather, it means that the body's estrogen production is not balanced by progesterone production. In other words, estrogen dominance begins to occur when the ovaries continue to produce the same amount of estrogen while they produce less and less progesterone. Estrogen dominance occurs when the natural ratio of estrogen to progesterone is upset. From their mid-thirties on, almost all women are estrogen dominant.

 Some of the more common symptoms of estrogen dominance include:

Weight Gain (Waist, Hips)	Heart Palpitations
Depression	Bone Loss
Osteoporosis	Sleep Disturbances
Mood Swings	Aches/Pains
Infertility	Fibromyalgia
Hot Flashes	Allergies
Low Sex Drive	Sensitivity to Chemicals
Fluid Retention	Stress
Headaches	Cold Body Temperature
Hair Loss	Sugar Craving
Fatigue	Elevated Triglycerides
Pre-Menstrual Syndrome (PMS)	Increased Facial/Body Hair
Fibrocystic Disease	Acne
Insomnia	Tender Breasts
Night Sweats	Bleeding Changes
Vaginal Dryness	Nervous
Incontinence	Irritable
Foggy Thinking	Anxious
Memory Lapse	Uterine Fibroids
Tearful	Endometriosis
Depressed	Candida

Peri-menopause literally means around menopause. This transition phase can last anywhere from two to eight years; however, women in this lifecycle are typically late forties to early fifties. Their ovaries are still producing eggs although ovulation may be occurring irregularly. They are at a late reproductive stage of their lives and it is still possible to conceive. These are the years when an occasional couple who has grown children in college suddenly discovers that they are going to have an "uh-oh" baby to bless the second phase of their lives. During peri-menopause, the ovaries continue to produce hormones but progesterone production declines even more significantly.

A woman is not officially menopausal until she has not had a period for at least twelve months. The average age of women entering natural menopause in the United States is fifty-one. Menopause, or "the change," marks the end of the reproductive years. The pituitary gland and the hypothalamus continue to produce their hormones (e.g. GnRH, FSH, and LH) but the ovaries are no longer able to produce enough estrogen to ovulate.

An uninformed medical community continues to treat menopause as an age-related disease, like high blood pressure or Alzheimer's. It is not a disease but a natural transition from one lifecycle to another. Many physicians also have the misconception that, once a woman enters menopause, her ovaries turn off like a light switch and stop producing all hormones. This is not true. In fact, the ovaries of a menopausal woman are still quite actively producing between forty to sixty percent of the estrogen and testosterone produced by a pre-menopausal woman. Progesterone production, however, continues to decline. At menopause, the continued decline in progesterone can lead to vaginal dryness, hot flashes, hair loss, and night sweats, as well as depression and mood swings.

Experiencing Sudden Shock: Hysterectomy and Artificial Menopause

Approximately one in every four American women will enter an abrupt, artificial menopause. The condition known as surgical menopause is the result of a complete hysterectomy. A hysterectomy is the option that most physicians commonly recommend for women who have fibroid tumors, severe endometriosis, cancer and/or constant, heavy bleeding. A complete hysterectomy involves surgical removal of the entire reproductive tract, including the uterus, tubes, and ovaries. Unfortunately, up to 90 percent of the time, a woman's pelvic organs will be removed for benign disease that could have been treated by non-surgical approaches.

Once a woman has had a complete hysterectomy, her body will immediately enter menopause regardless of her biological age. It is important to note that after a complete hysterectomy there are no ovaries to produce any level of hormones. As a result, the body goes into a kind of shock. Too many physicians make the common mistake of prescribing only estrogen for women after a complete hysterectomy, but estrogen alone is not enough. In fact, estrogen alone can foster a condition called **estrogen dominance**: when this occurs, it can be very dangerous to the body. After a complete hysterectomy, a women's body will need a new and balanced supply of all her sex hormones: estrogen, progesterone and testosterone.

The thought that the ovaries' production of hormones will not be affected by a partial hysterectomy (e.g. removal of the uterus only) is another common error in thinking made by too many physicians. The ovaries are significantly impacted because there are two primary pathways for blood flow to the ovaries: one is through the aorta and the second is through the uterus. When the uterus is removed, the flow of blood to the ovaries lessens, and consequently, the production of hormones is reduced. While the hormone imbalance may not be as great as with a complete hysterectomy, women who have a partial hysterectomy should be tested and treated to ensure optimal hormone balance.

Artificial menopause can also occur as a result of radiation or chemotherapy, or by the administration of certain drugs that catalyze menopause for medical reasons (such as to shrink fibroid tumors). Because there is no opportunity for gradual adjustment to the hormonal drop-off, the symptoms of artificial menopause can be sudden, severe and debilitating: requiring a more immediate intervention of supplemental hormone therapy.

After menopause, the ovaries continue to produce a significant amount of testosterone. In fact, the production of testosterone continues long after the ovaries have significantly decreased their production of both progesterone and estrogen. Is there such a thing as testosterone dominance? Absolutely! Have you ever encountered an older woman with more than a little facial hair and a particularly gruff or deep sounding voice? Odds are that she was suffering from having too much testosterone within her system.

Please note that the age ranges listed with the above lifecycles are not absolute indicators. For instance, a thirty-eight year old woman who has not had a period for fourteen months could be menopausal. Similarly, there are women in their late forties and early fifties who should have been finished with the reproductive years but whose ovaries continued to produce enough estrogen for them to ovulate and conceive. Ultimately, it will be the hormonal activity of a woman's ovaries - not her age - that defines which lifecycle she is in.

Chapter 2

Introducing a Circle of Women.... and Men

It should now be obvious that the issues associated with hormone balance should **not** be relegated to middle-aged women going through "the change." Every woman's body and hormone balance will change with age, and no matter what lifecycle she might presently be in, every woman's hormones will play a key role in dictating physical, mental and emotional health as well as quality of life.

Once you understand how important it is to support your body's natural hormonal equilibrium, you can be more confident in taking an active role with your physician to determine the best medical option for addressing your individual concerns. Again, no matter what your age and current hormonal state, knowledge of the issues at hand can provide you with both choice and insight. Women come to see me because they have something going on "in there" that is causing them real physical discomfort and/or emotional distress. While their ages and presenting symptoms may differ significantly, most of them share a common concern: they all suffer from hormone imbalance. Between my four nurse practitioners and myself, we see approximately one hundred and fifty patients per week. We recognize that each patient is an individual and we listen to both her stories and her body as we strive to find a safe and effective solution for her concerns.

My patients tell me that it can be both tedious and overwhelming to wade through a bunch of medical terminology and biochemical formulas trying to grasp what is going on with their hormones and their choices regarding hormone therapies. They ask me to give them medical information and advice in plain language. Often wanting to learn from real-life examples, patients probe me to find out what has and hasn't worked for other women who had similar symptoms.

I am adamant that there is no "one-size-fits-all" approach to hormone therapy. Every human body has its own specific make up. For example, all diabetics don't take the same dose of insulin. Why would we think that all women suffering from hormonal imbalances take the same dosage of ovarian hormones?

While physicians need to evaluate each female patient to determine her individual hormonal ratios and concerns, the following five case studies are representative of some of the most frequently occurring scenarios and symptoms associated with hormone imbalance. The names of these patients are ficticious. Perhaps you will recognize something of your own story as you read theirs.

Case Study #1: Carol / Heavy, Hot, and Angry At Forty-Seven Years Old

Upon entering my consultation office, I was greeted by Carol who immediately told me, "I want my life back." Carol went on to tell me that, starting about a year ago, at age forty-four, she began to occasionally skip periods. She said that sometimes she would be regular for four to five months and then would go three months without menstruating. "Then, when I do have a period," she reported, "it is so heavy that I flood for days."

"I can live with that, Dr. Randolph," she went on, "but it seems like I am on the verge of going through "the change" (menopause) and I am afraid that it will destroy my life and marriage." "How is that, Carol?" I asked, although I was pretty sure that I already had a good idea of what she was going to tell me. "Well," she replied, "first, I don't even like myself any more, so I sure as heck can understand why Dan, my husband, doesn't like me as much either. It seems like everything annoys me. Even when I am trying to be nice, I still seem to snap at everyone these days. I listen to myself and I know I must sound like a shrew in a bad movie."

"Also, I look old, really old, and it just seemed to happen overnight," she continued. "My hair seems to be falling out by the handful. I look in the mirror and I wonder where that fat woman with sagging skin came from. I've gained weight around my middle that, no matter how I work out or starve myself, just won't budge. Then, one day last month my nine year old son looked at me and said, "Mom, how come your face is falling down?" I couldn't help myself; I went in the bathroom and cried and cried."

"Finally," Carol confided, "Dan and I don't sleep in the same bedroom anymore. He says it is because I am always so hot and throwing off the covers. He started wearing pajamas but said that even with those on he froze and kept catching colds." Here she stopped and blushed, "I mean, Dr. Randolph, up until a few years ago we both slept naked. I started wearing nightgowns because I was ashamed of how heavy I had gotten." Carol whispered as she told me, "We used to have a lovely intimate relationship but now we hardly touch anymore."

"Oh, for heavens sake," Carol stormed as she threw up her hands, "If this is what the rest of my life is going to be like, just shoot me now!"

If she hadn't seemed so genuinely frustrated, I might have chuckled because her story was a variation of ones I had heard many times before. Instead, I took her hand in mine and said, "For now, Carol, let's leave the shotgun in the closet. I have some other ideas of what we might try first."

Case Study #2: Natalie / Fifty-Three and Feeling Like She Was "Falling Apart"

Natalie began crying the minute I opened the exam room door. "Dr. Randolph," she gulped, "I hope you can help me. I think I must have early Alzheimer's and everything else in my body is going wrong too." As a gynecologist, you wouldn't think I'd be the physician of choice to consult about early senility but I actually hear this complaint many times in a week. Memory problems can be symptomatic of hormone imbalance. Given her age and the fact that she had entered menopause two years prior at fifty-one years of age, I guessed that Natalie was right to consult me and I began to ask her some questions.

"I want to talk about your concerns regarding Alzheimer's disease, Natalie, but first tell me more about what else is going on with your body," I said. "What other concerns have brought you to see me?"

Natalie went on to tell me that she constantly felt as if something was pressing on her bladder and that she "peed when she sneezed." "Also," Natalie told me, "I look pregnant. I have always been a big girl but I have never had a stomach that sticks out like this. I guess it is because I retain so much fluid. Because I already feel as if I have to pee all the time, I don't want to take a diuretic. If I did, I am afraid that I would never be able to get out of the bathroom."

I asked Natalie if she had any problems with vaginal dryness and she said, "How would I know? I have been divorced for five years and no one goes visiting 'down there' any more." She quickly added, "Not that I really care. I never really go to bed anyway. Can't seem to sleep. I have decided that if I have my poodle, Charmin, and watch a movie in the middle of the night, I am much happier than when I had a man in my life!" I wondered about the truth of this statement but, for the time being, decided to focus on Natalie's gynecological rather than her social or emotional concerns.

Natalie shared with me that it had been the results of a bone density test that had prompted her to come see me. "I came to see you because I had this test at my previous gynecologist's office and the results said that I was suffering from significant bone loss. I am a golfer, Dr. Randolph, I can't become one of those stooped old women who shuffle around. I need my bones to be strong to carry me around to do what I want to do." With these last words, Natalie almost started to wail.

Natalie had given me a lot of information to work with but there was one more question I had to ask. "Natalie," I said, "why are you here to see me versus continuing to work with your previous gynecologist?"

"She (my gynecologist) wanted to prescribe Prempro, that estrogen drug made from horse urine." Natalie continued, "I don't know about all this synthetic versus natural hormone mumbo jumbo but I do know that I have a cousin who took that drug for years for her hot flashes and night sweats. My cousin was fifty-nine when she died last year of breast cancer. Before she passed over, she had started reading some articles that convinced her that that drug, Prempro, had in some way actually fed her cancer."

"My old doctor down played my concerns regarding Prempro's side effects," Natalie told me. "I heard from some friends that you take a more natural approach: working with women and prescribing some kind of human-identical hormones. I thought that you might help me find a safer alternative. Can you?"

"Natalie," I told her, "I think maybe I can."

Case Study #3: Barbara and Bob / Frightened, Lonely, and Helpless

I got a call from Bob one day asking for a phone consultation. He had concerns about his wife, Barbara, who at forty-one years old had had a complete hysterectomy because of fibroid tumors. "Now, two years later," he confided, "Barbara is so depressed that she almost seems like a zombie. She gets up, goes to work and comes home so tired that she just curls up on the couch and doesn't move. We used to come home and cook dinner together and talk and laugh the whole time." "Now," he continued, "if I try to talk to Barbara or persuade her to get up and go out and just do something fun, all she does is cry."

"Barbara will sometimes go through the motions and have sex with me, but I know that she does it more out of guilt than desire. Honestly, Dr. Randolph," Bob went on, "the sex isn't what it used to be. I mean, Barbara says her breasts are so tender that she doesn't want me to touch her there. Also, maybe because of that surgery Barbara had, intercourse isn't that easy. I once brought home some lubricant to see if that might help, but when Barbara saw it she just cried even more and said that I should just go ahead and trade her in for a younger model."

"The doctor that performed Barbara's surgery has her on some drug that I think is supposed to be replacing estrogen in her body. Whatever it is supposed to do, it is not working well enough. I was in your Natural Medicine Shoppe the other day buying vitamins and there was a TV running a video of you talking about some of the symptoms of hormone imbalance," Bob told me. "Maybe I am just grasping at straws but some of the things you were saying sounded like what Barbara has been going through. I also learned some new information, like the fact that because Barbara's body isn't producing all the hormones it used to, she could be at higher risk for bone loss and heart disease."

"Dr. Randolph, I know you must think I am some sort of goon because I have mostly talked about how our sex life has changed since Barbara had a hysterectomy. I love my wife and I will do anything I can to help her live a long, healthy, happy life. I miss our times together but, even more, I miss the woman I know must still be in there," Bob told me. "Can you help us?"

I told Bob that both he and Barbara have hope. I asked him to share my video on human-identical hormone therapies with Barbara. "Bob, I can only speak in general terms until I have both examined Barbara and reviewed the results of her individual hormone profile. If Barbara agrees, have her give my nurse a call and we will set up an office visit as soon as possible."

When I hung up, I thought of the courage it took for Bob to call up a gynecologist and try and find help for his wife. My heart went out to him and to Barbara. I sincerely hoped that I would have a chance to meet Barbara in the near future.

Case Study #4: Beth / A Superstar with Headaches, Fatigue, and a Low Sex Drive

When she first scheduled an appointment with our office, Beth said she just needed to come in for her annual check up. Beth reported that the OB/GYN she had previously been seeing had retired about a year ago and that, since she was an "informed consumer," she knew the importance of getting regular pap smears and mammograms. She said she had chosen our practice because, "It is located between my office and my children's day care. I can leave work early and still be on time to pick up my kids at the end of the day."

Beth was a model of efficiency and, on her first visit,

came prepared with copies of her past medical records. "Just the usual," she said as she handed her file to me. "I am thirty-six years old and I am glad to say that every thing stills seems to be in working order. After trying for several years, my husband and I were blessed enough three years ago to have twins, a boy and a girl." Beth sort of smiled and tucked a stray strand of perfectly coiffed hair behind her ear as she said, "Everyone laughed and said it was just like me to find an express lane for delivering a one-stop family!"

 "Anyway," she continued, "I always hated taking the pill so Rick (my husband) stepped up to the plate and got a vasectomy after the twins were born. Now, I'm as regular as clockwork." Beth shrugged a bit and then added, "Not that all that really matters. I am so exhausted when I go to bed that sex is the last thing I want to think about." I asked Beth a few more questions and learned that in addition to her tiredness and little interest in sex, she also frequently suffered from migraines. Beth attributed her fatigue, decreased libido and headaches to her schedule. Beth mentioned that she had pretty bad PMS (pre-menstrual syndrome) but, she said, "What woman who still has periods doesn't have PMS?"

Beth went on to explain that, in addition to being the mother of three-year-old twins, she was also a vice president of a successful public relations agency. She explained that she and her husband traded off taking the children to day care and picking them up. "Rick is in charge of mornings. I typically leave the house about 5 a.m. so that I can get my work done and not feel guilty about leaving at 4:30 p.m. to pick up the children. When I get home, I take charge of making dinner and giving the children their baths so Rick can have his time to work out."

"Dr. Randolph," she said, "I may not like the way I feel but it is understandable, don't you think? I mean I hate the way I act out with PMS every month but I get through it and," she added with a sort of sad wry smile, "so does my husband. With regard to my other symptoms - the fatigue, low sex drive and headaches - I guess I would feel better if I could figure out how to take a nap in the middle of the day but, really, I don't have that option. There really isn't anything that medical science could do to make me feel better, is there?"

"Actually, Beth," I replied, "there very well might be."

Case Study #5: Toni / A Young, Athletic Vegetarian Who Stopped Menstruating

Toni was twenty years old when she first came to see me. In our initial conversation, Toni tilted her chin defiantly upward and crossed her legs with intention as she informed me: "There is nothing wrong with me. I am only here to get my mother off my back. I have just finished my sophomore year of college and am about to transfer to from Florida State University to the University of California. I think my mother just wants to find something wrong with me so she can convince me to stay closer to home."

Toni had begun to menstruate at fifteen years of age and had regular periods until she was eighteen and entered college. For the next two years, her periods became increasingly irregular and finally just stopped. Her last period had been almost a year ago.

While Toni had an athletic look about her, she was too thin. Her weight, 107 lbs., was low for her five foot, six inch frame. When I asked Toni about her weight, she proudly told me that she was not one of those girls who gained the "freshmen ten pounds" in her first year of college and never lost it. In fact, she reported that when she first went to college she had been a bit "pudgy" and, as a result, had joined both a track and tennis team to try and work off the extra pounds. It had worked; she lost 14 lbs. over nine months. When I asked Toni about her diet, she proudly told me that she "ate very healthily and was a vegetarian."

In medical terms, an absence of menstruation is called **amenorrhea**. Toni believed that "it was no big deal" that she didn't menstruate regularly. "Actually," she said, "I am relieved that I don't have periods any more. They are just a big mess anyway." Despite Toni's satisfaction with her current state, I felt her mother was right in prodding her to come see me. It is not normal or healthy for a young woman of twenty years not to be menstruating regularly.

What Happens Next

Before a diagnosis could be made or treatment prescribed, each of the women in the previously described case studies needed to have a complete physical and an individualized hormone profile workup. Still, we can put to work some of the knowledge that you have gleaned from reading about a woman's endocrine system and her lifecycles.

With the data we have regarding their symptoms and ages, we can begin to make some educated guesses. The following table captures what we know so far.

Case Study	Age	Presenting Symptom(s)	Red Flags: Endocrine System Malfunctioning	Lifecycle	Preliminary Diagnosis
Carol	47	Irregular Periods Irritability Weight Gain Hair Loss Loss of Skin Tone Hot Flashes Night Sweats	Given Carol's age, irregular periods usually signal that <u>ovarian production of estrogen is</u> beginning to <u>decline</u> but <u>progesterone production will be declining even more.</u>	Peri-Menopause	Estrogen Dominant
Natalie	53	No Periods For Two Years. Memory Loss Urinary Incontinence Abdominal Bloating Insomnia Loss Of Interest In Sex Osteoporosis	Ovaries still producing some estrogen but not enough to foster a menstrual cycle. Progesterone production continues to decline and the consequent imbalance is great enough to cause a multiplicity of physical, mental and emotional symptoms.	Natural Menopause	Estrogen Dominant

Case Study	Age	Presenting Symptom(s)	Red Flags: Endocrine System Malfunctioning	Lifecycle	Preliminary Diagnosis
Barbara (and Bob)	43	Severe Depression Fibrocystic Breasts Vaginal Dryness	The surgical removal of Barbara's uterus, cervix, tubes and ovaries has stripped her of critical key organs for hormonal support. Most likely, Barbara's system is suffering from a kind of shock stemming from insufficient hormone production. Abrupt cessation of natural hormone production is usually much more severe than with a gradual peri-menopausal decline. The fact that Barbara's gynecologist had placed her on some form of synthetic estrogen without addressing the fact that her body was also now lacking in progesterone and testosterone actually fosters estrogen dominance.	Surgical Menopause	Estrogen Dominant

Case Study	Age	Presenting Symptom(s)	Red Flags: Endocrine System Malfunctioning	Lifecycle	Preliminary Diagnosis
Beth	36	Extreme Fatigue PMS Low Libido Migraines	Extreme fatigue may be a signal that the <u>adrenal gland</u> function is compromised. Because Beth has a regular menstrual cycle, her <u>ovaries are most likely maintaining a constant production of estrogen</u>; however, the other symptoms (e.g. PMS, low libido and migraines) probably indicate that Beth's <u>ovarian production of progesterone has begun to drop off.</u>	Pre-Menopause	Estrogen Dominant Adrenal Exhaustion
Toni	20	Absence of Periods (Amenorrhea) Body Weight Too Low	Vegetarian diet and low body weight mean that the body <u>probably is lacking sufficient cholesterol: the building block molecule for all hormone production.</u> Insufficient hormone production will impede the function of entire endocrine system. Toni's <u>pituitary and hypothalamus glands</u> are most likely <u>not producing enough GnRH, FSH, and LH</u> to stimulate the rise of estrogen and progesterone during her monthly cycle. The <u>ovaries are probably not producing enough estrogen to regulate periods.</u>	Early Reproductive Years	Hypo-Estrogenic Amenorrhea

At any age and for any reason, when a woman's natural hormonal equilibrium is altered, she will require some form of hormone replacement therapy to restore hormone balance. What are the options?

In the next two chapters, we will examine the controversy currently raging in the medical community regarding the safety and efficacy of synthetic hormone replacement therapies (HRT) versus human-identical hormones.

Chapter 3

Synthetic Hormone Replacement Therapy (HRT): A Pharmaceutical "Dr. Jekyll and Mr. Hyde"

Once you understand how hormone balance shifts with age, you can also recognize how hormone imbalance can be the underlying issue for many physical, emotional and mental concerns. It would seem obvious that reinstating your body's original hormonal ratios could potentially alleviate the unpleasant symptoms and support optimal health. In other words, if you replace what is missing, your body will work better.

Hormone replacement really is a pretty simple concept. Unfortunately, most of the medical community is still having trouble grasping it. Because I know that the majority of my physician peers are intelligent and caring patient advocates, I assign most of the blame to the pharmaceutical industry. I believe that big drug companies have twisted and manipulated the idea of hormone replacement to capitalize on a business opportunity.

Synthetic hormone replacement therapies (HRT) began development in the 1940s. By the 1970s, HRT was almost a household word. Nature dictated that women would sooner or later suffer the unwanted symptoms typically associated with menopause. It did not take sophisticated market research for the pharmaceutical industry to recognize that they would have female customers waiting-in-the-wings if products could be developed.

Over several decades, the pharmaceutical industry instigated a bonanza of press releases touting synthetic HRT as the female fountain of youth. Dollars and manpower were committed to tapping into a market niche of approximately 38.5 million baby-boomer women now entering their 40's and 50's. From a business perspective, the pharmaceutical industry has been successful. In 2002, synthetic HRT was used by 38 percent of women suffering from menopausal symptoms.

Unfortunately, it seems as if the drug companies have created a pharmaceutical version of Dr. Jekyll and Mr. Hyde. If you remember the plot from Robert Louis Stevenson's classic horror tale, Dr. Jekyll had the appearance of a kind and respected physician who healed and cared for people. The plot went on to reveal that Dr. Jekyll had a dangerous double nature. His tormented psyche took the name of Mr. Hyde who was capable of performing gruesome acts, including murder. Once exposed, neither Dr. Jekyll nor Mr. Hyde could survive.

The metaphor here is potent. Like Dr. Jekyll, synthetic HRT made a good first impression. When the pharmaceutical industry originally launched synthetic HRT formulations, physicians were enthusiastic about finally having a product that they could prescribe to alleviate their patients' symptoms associated with hormone imbalance and menopause. Initially, the female patients they placed on these synthetic HRT drugs were ecstatic to have relief for symptoms like hot flashes, vaginal dryness and night sweats. These women felt that they had been given a medical miracle that would help them more gracefully navigate their "change of life."

Over the last several years, however, a Mr. Hyde phenomenon has been shadowing the original popularity of synthetic HRT. The double nature of synthetic HRT has been exposed. We are experiencing an initial crescendo of mounting clinical evidence that synthetic HRT should not be taken long-term because it manifests more chronic health risks than short-term benefits.

Given the evidence, the pharmaceutical industry's ongoing efforts to convince physicians to prescribe new variations of synthetic HRT is almost criminal. The most critical issues include the following:

1. For the last 50+ years, the pharmaceutical industry has focused on developing 'one-size-fits-all' synthetic HRT products. For the most part, they have ignored that each woman's body has a genetically predetermined hormone balance directing the interaction of all her sex hormones (e.g. estrogen, progesterone, testosterone).

2. While the pharmaceutical industry originally mass-marketed synthetic hormone HRT as a panacea for relief of hot flashes, vaginal dryness, protection from osteoporosis and cardiovascular disease, recent clinical studies have shown that HRT can be more harmful than helpful and can actually foster many long-term, and *potentially terminal* health concerns.

3. The pharmaceutical industry has misinformed physicians. If big drug companies were truly patient advocates, they would use their extensive research facilities and large field sales forces to educate the medical community about hormone testing and natural or human-identical hormone therapies. Of course from a business perspective, the dollar opportunity for the pharmaceutical

industry is exponentially greater when they can promote and nationally distribute a standard HRT product to physicians and chain pharmacies. As I will discuss later, human-identical hormones cannot be patented. As a result, when a physician writes an individualized prescription for a patient that is then compounded (made from scratch) in a compounding pharmacy, there is relatively little financial gain for pharmaceutical companies.

A Business Opportunity: Pharmaceutical Hype and Spin

Synthetic hormone compounds have chemical molecules that have been forceably joined together via laboratory synthesis. In the medical literature discussing HRT, the terms "conjugated" and "synthetic" are often used interchangeably. Another term that you might see is "exogenous hormones," meaning hormones produced outside the human body. From a business perspective, it is important that synthetic hormone compounds can be patented, thereby giving the pharmaceutical company manufacturer exclusive ownership of both the chemical formula and the revenue the patented product generates for a period of time.

Don't get confused or intimidated by the chemical language. What you need to know is simply that none of the estrogen compounds manufactured by the pharmaceutical industry have the same molecular structure as the hormones produced by the human ovaries. The issues associated with the synthetic formulation of the molecular structure of naturally occurring hormones will soon be explained but, for now, let's return and examine the market trajectory of synthetic HRTs.

In 1949, Wyeth-Ayerst Pharmaceuticals first introduced Premarin, a drug composed of conjugated estrogenic compounds. Premarin is the brand name for equinal which is derived from the urine of pregnant mares. By the early 1970's, Premarin was regarded as the medical "gold standard" for treating menopausal symptoms such as hot flashes, vaginal dryness and atrophy, depression and low libido. For several years, Wyeth-Ayerst capitalized on the HRT market niche and relished its position as a pharmaceutical leader in the women's health market. Then in 1975, medical evidence caused the pharmaceutical giant to fumble. Clinical studies reported a link between synthetic horse estrogen and uterine (endometrial) cancer.

As a result of the clinical evidence, the FDA took a first stand. Wyeth-Ayerst was required to include the warning as a package insert with every prescription (see next page). You would have thought that with these kinds of serious side effects, Premarin would have been pulled off the market. Sales did decline for awhile but the pharmaceutical industry was not about to walk away from a billion dollar market opportunity. The big drug companies took a different tactic.

The term "unopposed estrogen" was coined. Estrogen was known to stimulate the growth of estrogen-sensitive tissue, such as the tissue found in the uterus and the breast. Wyeth-Ayerst and other pharmaceutical companies acknowledged that too much estrogen could have a

> ## Official Premarin Warning Label
> **Estrogens Have Been Reported To Increase the Risk of Endometrial Carcinoma**
>
> Three independent, case-controlled studies have reported an increased risk of endometrial cancer in post-menopausal women exposed to exogenous estrogens for more than one year. The risk was independent of the other known risk factors for endometrial cancer. These studies are further reported by the finding that incidence rates of endometrial cancer have increased sharply since 1969 in eight different areas of the United States with population-based cancer-reporting systems, an increase that may be related to the rapidly expanding use of estrogens during the last decade.
>
> The three case-controlled studies reported that the risk of endometrial cancer in estrogen users was about 4.5 to 13.9 times greater than in nonusers.
>
> Source: Wyeth-Ayerst product package insert

carcinogenic affect. Their premise was that this concern could be eliminated if the estrogen was balanced with progesterone. These pharmaceutical companies synthesized a version of human progesterone and labeled it "progestin" or Provera.

Like the synthetic estrogens, the synthetic progesterone "progestin" was not identical to the progesterone produced by the human body. However, the pharmaceutical giants contended that these synthetic versions that they could patent and make a profit on were good enough. In fact, several clinical studies seemed to indicate that uterine (endometrial) cancer could actually be prevented if Provera (a brand name of progestin) was prescribed along with equinal (horse estrogen) found in Premarin.

With the help of marketing promotions and rallying pharmaceutical sales forces, combination synthetic estrogen-progestin HRT became the new cure-all. Wyeth-Ayerst recognized the advent of synthetic combination HRT as yet another opportunity and, over the next few years, launched two conjugated estrogen/medroxyprogesterone tablets (e.g. Prempro and Premphase). In addition to addressing menopausal symptoms like hot flashes and night sweats while also preventing uterine cancer, these drugs were endowed with a medical halo that included preventing osteoporosis and cardiac concerns while even warding off Alzheimer's disease. For decades, the medical community bought into all the hype and readily prescribed the synthetic HRT drugs for their patients complaining of the symptoms of hormone imbalance.

In both her book *The Hormone Solution, Two Scientific Studies* (published in 1998) and in her work published in 1999 in *Chemical Research and Toxicology and Proceedings of the Society for Biological Medicine*, Dr. Erika Schwartz proved that once broken down in our bodies, conjugated equine estrogen (e.g. Premarin) becomes toxic to the very DNA that keeps us healthy or makes us sick. By 2002, Wyeth-Ayerst's top-selling synthetic HRT drugs accounted for approximately 70 million prescriptions and $1 billion in yearly sales revenue.

The Women's Health Initiative Study: The Horror Is Revealed

In 1993, the National Institutes of Health (NIH) initiated a drug trial know as the Women's Health Initiative (WHI). The overall objective of this study was to explore the effects of synthetic combination estogren-progestin HRT on the long-term health of menopausal women. The study was intended to run until 2005 but was stopped after an average follow up of only 5.2 years. It involved 16,608 healthy women between the ages of 50 and 79 with an intact uterus (none of these women had had a hysterectomy prior to entering the study). An important objective for the trial was to examine the effect of estrogen plus progestin on the prevention of heart disease and hip fractures, and any associated change in risk for breast and colon cancer. The study was not designed to address the short-term risks and benefits of hormones for the treatment of menopausal symptoms.

Participants were enrolled in the study between 1993 and 1998 at over 40 clinical sites across the country. Women enrolled in the study were randomly assigned to a daily dose of estrogen plus progestin (0.625 mg of conjugated equine estrogens plus 2.5 mg of medroxyprogesterone acetate), also known by the brand name Prempro. Half the women were given the Prempro, while the rest received a sugar pill placebo. Wyeth-Ayerst donated the Prempro.

In 2000 and 2001, WHI investigators complied with a recommendation from the study's Data and Safety Monitoring Board (DSMB) to inform participants of a small increase in heart attacks, strokes and blood clots in women taking the synthetic hormones. The DSMB, an independent advisory committee charged with reviewing results and ensuring participant safety, found that the actual number of women having any one of these events did not cross the statistical boundary established to ensure participant safety. Therefore, in both 2000 and 2001, the group recommended continuing the trial as they felt that the balance of risks and benefits was still uncertain.

Almost simultaneously, a separate government scientific advisory panel was formed and charged with analyzing the link between synthetic HRT and cancer. In 2001, this panel of experts published an opinion that dramatically contrasted with the DSMB's decision to continue the WHI study. Representatives from the National Cancer Institute and the NIH voted 8-1 to add synthetic estrogen to the nation's list of cancer causing agents.

Not long after, at the DSMB's regularly scheduled meeting on May 31, 2002, the data from the WHI study revealed

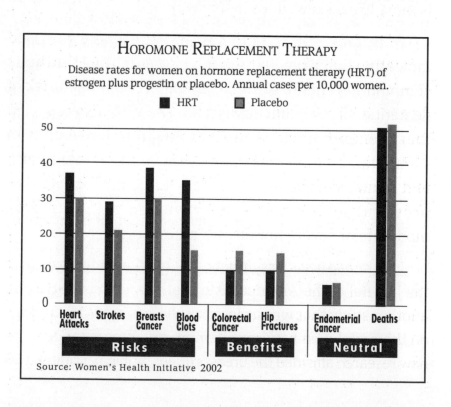

that the number of invasive breast cancers had crossed the established signal for risk. Consequently, the WHI study was abruptly halted in July 2002. The initial findings showed that women taking synthetic combination HRT (e.g. Prempro) had an increased risk of heart disease, breast cancer, stroke and blood clots. The study projected that for every 10,000 women taking on synthetic combination HRT (e.g. Prempro) there would be seven more coronary heart disease events, eight more breast cancers and eight more strokes than for 10,000 women taking nothing or a placebo. It is important to note that between 30 to 35 percent of the women originally enrolled in the study dropped out due to fear and/or side effects. Consequently, the number of women projected to suffer potentially critical side effects is most likely skewed to the low end.

In May 2003, additional findings were released indicating that women over 65 who were taking synthetic combination HRT (e.g. Prempro) had a heightened risk of dementia, or Alzheimer's disease. The WHI also reported that Prempro provided no meaningful improvement in such quality-of-life measures as sleep, emotional health and sexual satisfaction. The study did find that Prempro provided some relief among women suffering from moderate or severe hot flashes and/or night sweats.

The bad news for synthetic HRT continued. In June 2003, the Journal of the American Medical Association published another study that was a closer analysis of the WHI findings on the correlation between Prempro and breast cancer. The new research affirmed the breast cancer problem, finding a 26 percent increase in the risk of breast cancer for women taking the synthetic HRT formulation. In addition, the report from the Harbor-UCLA Research and Education Institute found that the cancers tend to be diagnosed at more advanced stages and result in substantial increases in abnormal mammograms. The report of increased risk was not reported with the first findings. Although the breast tumors were most likely already present, they were not detected because the hormone drugs caused increased breast density. This means that when the women were on Prempro, tumors in their breasts were harder to find. Consequently, when these tumors were detected, the cancer was more advanced.

In the same time frame, a study appeared in the *Journal of the National Cancer Institute* in which Swedish researchers reported that women using synthetic estrogen replacement therapy had a 43 percent increased risk of ovarian cancer. The study went on to report that those women on a combination of synthetic estrogen and progestin had a 54 percent increased risk of ovarian cancer.

A Lot or a Little Poison

Despite the halt of the study analyzing the benefits and drawbacks of synthetic combination HRT, there is branch of the WHI clinical trial that is continuing to study the effects of synthetic estrogen alone. This is of great concern to me. Synthetic estrogen is listed as a carcinogenic agent: what more evidence does the WHI need to halt current clinical trials? Can the medical community not simply reflect back to the earlier studies citing the carcinogenic effects of Wyeth-Ayerst's original synthetic estrogen only drug, Premarin? Why do physicians need to repeat past mistakes? Do we need new studies, and the wasting of more lives, to disprove the brainwashing that the pharmaceutical industry has subjected us to?

Unfortunately, even after the findings of the WHI study were released, many physicians continue to express surprise

---

The Evidence

June 2003: Breast cancer in women taking combination synthetic estrogen-progestin HRT may be harder to detect and more aggressive when found; findings from an analysis of the government's landmark WHI study.

May 2003: Combination synthetic estrogen-progestin HRT linked to doubling the risk of Alzheimer's disease and other forms of dementia in older women; from another analysis of the WHI data.

January 2003: The FDA requires that the highest level of warning information in labeling be included with every prescription of synthetic estrogen or estrogen-progestin HRT. The label highlights the increased risks for heart disease, strokes and breast cancer.

July 2002: The WHI study of more than 16,000 women links combination synthetic estrogen-progestin HRT pills to an increased risk of breast cancer, heart attack and strokes.

January 2001: A Seattle HMO study of 5,212 postmenopausal women finds increased breast density in those taking synthetic HRT.

2001: A government scientific advisory panel votes to add synthetic estrogen to the nation's list of carcinogenic agents

2001: A study appears in the Journal of the National Cancer Institute linking synthetic estrogen as well as synthetic estrogen + progestin to a significant rise in the risk of ovarian cancer.

Source: *International Position Paper on Women's Health And Menopuase: A Comprehensive Approach. National Heart, Blood and Lung Institute. July 2002.*

---

over the negative outcomes. Others have tried to completely ignore or gloss over the clinical evidence showing that the synthetic HRT drugs they were in the habit of prescribing could actually be harmful to their patients.

Why are these drugs still the most commonly prescribed treatment for the negative symptoms associated with hormone imbalance and menopause? Why are doctors today still prescribing these synthetic pharmaceutical products that could significantly harm rather than help their patients? With all the scientific and clinical evidence available today regarding the health risks of synthetic HRT, I contend that it is almost criminal for physicians to continue to plead ignorance and as a result, prescribe synthetic hormones that have been clinically proven to be carcinogenic. In the past, many physicians were truly brainwashed regarding the benefits of synthetic HRT. Today, however, I believe that some of my physician peers remain legitimately confused by the contradictory evidence in the medical literature and continuing education programs. Others, unfortunately, prefer to remain in a state of denial.

In 2002, Adriane Fugh-Berman, M.D., and Cynthia Pearson, B.A., published an article in Pharmacotherapy Publications entitled "The Overselling of Hormone Replacement Therapy." In this article, the authors addressed the most potent issue at hand: "Why did the medical and research community ever believe that synthetic HRT prevented or treated disease?" They cited research evidence that revealed not a single controlled trial had ever demonstrated any positive disease prevention benefits of synthetic HRT.

The pharmaceutical industry launched aggressive marketing campaigns to convince physicians that synthetic HRT could prevent many chronic concerns, including cardiovascular disease. How did the pharmaceutical industry get away with this? What caused the medical community to suspend its usual requirement for data from credible double-blind randomized controlled trials?

While advertising and the perks offered by many pharmeceutical sales representatives have had an impact on physicians' awareness and prescribing patterns, these were only a small part of the campaign. Far more effective was the hidden influence that the pharmaceutical industry had on the information physicians received through medical meetings and continuing medical education activities. For decades, these forums vehemently endorsed and espoused the benefits of synthetic HRT. How could this be? Well, remember that in most cases the pharmaceutical companies were footing the bill for the meetings and, as the old saying goes, money talks. No wonder

---

SYNTHETIC HORMONE BRAND NAMES

Premarin

Prempro

Premphase

Femhrt

Activella

Ortho-prefest

Combipatch

Cenestin

Menest

Ortho-est

Ogen

Estratab

WHAT IS "SYNTHETIC"?

"Patented" or "Conventional" or "Artificial"

Usually not found in nature or at least not in humans

Chemically altered form of human hormone

Not identical in structure or activity to natural hormones they try to emulate

most of the medical community still does not know what to believe about hormone replacement therapies. For years, their minds have been manipulated by the educational forums they were trained to trust.

Despite all the conflicting and alarmist scrutiny synthetic HRT has been under, the pharmaceutical industry is gearing up to launch marketing campaigns for lower dose or different formulation estrogen-progestin therapies. There are already some marketing efforts attempting to foster a resurgence of synthetic-estrogen-only therapies. Here are a few reasons to fear that, once again, the pharmaceutical companies marketing efforts could be successful:

- First, the market still exists. Female patients continue to clamor for relief and their doctors still want to help them.

- Secondly, in 2003, Wyeth-Ayerst won government approval to market lower doses of its synthetic estrogen-progestin combination HRT sold as Prempro.

- Thirdly, the pharmaceutical industry continues to be the top funder of specialty forums and continuing medical education meetings for doctors.

- Finally, the pharmaceutical industry offers physicians some nice "perks," such as lunches for office staff, dinners on the town, fishing trips and sports event tickets. Credible or questionable, the money the pharmaceutical companies spend wins them the ear of the physician.

As long as the pharmaceutical industry has an influence on medical education, physicians will be challenged to seek out information and teach themselves about the options and choices related to synthetic HRT versus human-identical hormone replacement therapies.

The tragedy is that tens of thousands of women are developing cancer because their physicians continue to allow themselves to be brainwashed. If the pharmaceutical companies took the high road and began to educate the physicians regarding the real clinical concerns associated with synthetic HRT, as well as what alternative therapies might be available, they would cannibalize a sizeable revenue stream. It really comes down to business dollars versus patient care.

Again, many of my physician peers are legitimately confused; others choose to remain ignorant. The good news is that the consumer may soon have more power than the pharmaceutical industry. As women read articles and watch TV shows about the output of the WHI study and the concerns associated with synthetic HRT, they realize that they may be faced with a difficult decision when it comes to symptoms versus treatment. They are looking for alternatives because an all or nothing scenario doesn't work for them. In many cases, women have chosen to leave their previous physicians because they could not get the information and support needed to make informed decisions. Many women come to see me because they know that I eschew the synthetic products and have a different approach that has been proven to work again and again.

When these women come into my office today, they don't look to me to be their "physician savior." They have already done their homework and researched their choices. They come armed with clinical studies and ask very informed questions. As their doctor, I find this very exciting. I also think it could be the saving grace for most of my physician peers.

Doctors don't want to lose their patients, but they will if they don't wake up. They can choose to educate themselves about more natural hormone treatment options, including human-identical hormone therapies. Of course, studies validating the safety and efficacy of these natural solutions won't be provided to doctors by pharmaceutical representatives. I think that this is a good thing. As physicians review the data and educate themselves without the influence of a business that is vested in directing prescribing patterns, they can better return to their role as an informed and objective patient advocate.

Smart, informed and demanding women are finding their voice and they want data that they can believe and trust. As more and more women educate themselves about alternatives and natural choices for hormone replacement, they will begin to demand that their physicians prescribe human-identical therapies as their treatment of choice. These informed women will become their own grass-roots sales force. Pharmaceutical representatives won't stand a chance. My hope is that across America women will create a groundswell of new awareness regarding the benefits of human-identical hormone therapies that the medical community will not be able to ignore. Perhaps the pharmaceutical companies' synthetic HRT potions will be unable to survive.

Hope on the Horizon: Biopharmaceutical Companies

I am gratified to report that, today, there are several specialty biopharmaceutical companies dedicating resources and dollars to developing proprietary human-identical/bio-identical hormone products. The following is a list of some of the products with which I am currently familiar and prescribe in my own practice. Each of these has been approved by the FDA.

Brand name: ***Estrasorb***
Mode of Delivery: Topical emulsion/transdermal
        application
Manufacturer: Novavax, Inc.
Marketed by: Novavax, Inc. Corporate Headquarters
      8320 Guilford Road, Suite C
      Columbia, Maryland 21046
      www.novavax.com

Brand name: ***EstroGel***
Mode of Delivery: Topical emulsion/transdermal
        application
Manufacturer: R. P. Scherger North America
Marketed by: Solvay Pharmaceuticals, Inc. Corporate
      Headquarters
      Marietta, Georgia 30062
      www.solvaypharmaceuticals.com

Brand name: ***Estrace***
Mode of Delivery: Estradiol tablets/oral adminstration
Manufacturer: Bristol-Myers Squibb Co.
Marketed by: Warner Chilcott, Inc.
> Rockaway, NJ 07866
> www.estrace.com

There are also many generic forms of estradiol on the market, as well as many estradiol skin "patches" currently available by prescription from a physician. It is also important to note that the product inserts for most of these products state that: "using human-identical estradiol products without human-identical progesterone may increase the risk of heart attacks, strokes, breast cancer and blood clots."

 Human-Identical Progesterone
Brand name: ***Crinone***
Mode of Delivery: Bioadhesive vaginal gel
Manufacturer: Serono, Inc.
Marketed by: Serono, Inc. Corporate Headquarters
> One Technology Place
> Rockland, Maryland 02370
> www.seronousa.com

Brand name: ***Prochieve***
Mode of Delivery: Bioadhesive vaginal gel
Manufacturer: Columbia Laboratories, Inc.
Marketed by: Columbia Laboratories, Inc.
> 354 Eisenhower Parkway
> Second Floor, Plaza 1
> Livingston, New Jersey 07039
> www.columbialabs.com

Brand name: ***Prometrium***
Mode of Delivery: Micronized progesterone in peanut oil/
                 capsules/oral administration
Manufacturer: R. P. Scherger North America
Marketed by: Solvay Pharmaceuticals, Inc. Corporate
                 Headquarters
                 Marietta, Georgia 30062
                 www.solvaypharmaceuticals.com

Human-Identical Testosterone
Brand name: ***Androgel***
Mode of Delivery: Testosterone gel/transdermal
                 application
Marketed by: Solvay Pharmaceuticals, Inc. Corporate
                 Headquarters
                 Marietta, Georgia 30062
                 www.androgel.com

Brand name: ***Testoderm***
Mode of Delivery: Skin patch
Manufacturer: ALZA Corporation
Marketed by: 1900 Charleston Road
                 Mountain View, California 94043
                 www.alza.com

Chapter 4

You Do Have a Choice

If you stopped reading this book right now, you would be like most of the women and physicians in the world today:

- frustrated by the symptoms of hormone imbalance,

- confused by the marketing hype from the pharmaceutical companies touting their latest and greatest product for menopausal symptoms, and

- frightened by the fact that the WHI study demonstrated that the use of synthetic HRT and horse estrogens results in more health risks than benefits.

The good news is that there are other options and you do have a choice. First, you can keep reading and learn about the benefits of human-identical hormone therapies. Then, bolstered with new information and knowledge, you can explore how these safe and effective treatment regimens for balancing your hormones can also protect your health and improve the quality of your life. You can also continue to read additional medical research about hormone replacement. Finally, you can ask your personal physician for his/her opinion. It is important to remember, however, that once you become an informed consumer you don't have to be victim to someone else's decision - even that of your doctor. You alone *can* and *should* have the final say when it comes to deciding which hormone replacement option is right for you.

Human-Identical Hormones: Keys That Fit

Within the body, hormones circulate within the bloodstream to all the tissues but they target only the cells that contain hormone receptor sites specific to that hormone. The hormones attach to these receptor sites like keys fitting into locks. The chemical term for this key and lock phenomenon is called **relative binding affinity**, or RBA. The hormones produced within the human body have a 100 percent RBA for their respective receptor sites.

The hormone key attaches to the receptor site for a purpose. Once the "fit" occurs, the body's cells can respond by carrying out their originally programmed hormonal functions. These functions will be specific to each hormone-receptor site pair. Problems begin to occur when the female body is no longer producing the optimum ratio of the "right" hormones for the "right" receptor sites.

In order for this lock and key metaphor to make sense, it may be helpful to review what you've learned so far. In Chapter 1, you read about how the endocrine system produces hormones. You also learned how the hormones produced within the endocrine system serve as chemical messengers that control such biological activities as menstruation, reproduction, growth, development, stress response, libido, metabolism and energy.

Chapter 1 also included data to evidence how hormone production and hormone balance changes with age. It explained how these shifts in hormonal ratios mean that often there aren't enough of the "right" hormones to attach to their respective receptor sites. You learned that when the lock and key ratio is upset, optimum biological performance becomes compromised, causing such common symptoms as hot flashes, mood swings, irregular bleeding, bloating, headaches, vaginal dryness, weight gain, low libido and premature aging.

Chapter 1 then concluded with the introduction of a "circle of women...and men." You read how each woman suffered from symptoms associated with hormone imbalance. As their stories unfolded, you were witness to the fact that while these women were of all ages and had various complaints, they shared common concerns. To some degree, they all felt victimized by their hormone changes. In addition, they all wanted some form of medical treatment to relieve their symptoms and get them back to "normal." Finally, many of these women were frightened by what they had heard and read about synthetic hormones. They were confused about their options for safe and effective hormone replacement. As you read about these women you could see how they might characterize the concerns, fears and questions of most women, if not yourself.

In Chapter 2, you saw how the pharmaceutical industry has built a huge business around targeting women just like the circle of women described in Chapter 1. You read how these companies have capitalized on treating menopausal symptoms by patenting formulations of synthetic hormones and aggressively marketing synthetic HRT to the medical community. You also learned that, in the last few years, research has shown that synthetic HRT can significantly increase a woman's risk of heart disease, breast cancer, stroke and blood clots, not to mention endometriosis, fibrocystic disease of the breast, and uterine fibroids. You were made aware that while the mass-market penetration of synthetic HRT generated billions of dollars for these pharmaceutical companies, many women suffered unduly in the process.

The concept of replacing what was missing sounded good enough, but instead of proving to be a safe and effective solution for women suffering from the symptoms of hormone imbalance, synthetic HRT actually unlocked doors leading to many health dangers. What went so wrong with synthetic HRT? Very simply, synthetic hormones are not an exact fit for the human body's hormone receptor sites; they are not the right key for the lock.

Because they are molecularly different in structure than the hormones they were designed to replace, synthetic hormones act as a foreign substance within the human body. As a result, their effects are not consistent with the body's normal biochemistry. The fact that synthetic HRT has been found to cause many unpredictable and harmful side effects comes down to a single fact: when it comes to replicating the biochemistry of the human body, *almost* the same molecular structure is not good enough.

In contrast, human-identical hormones have a molecular structure that exactly matches the molecular structure of the hormones produced by the female body. This means that, when human-identical hormones enter the bloodstream, they look and perform just like the original hormones they were designed to replicate. Human-identical hormones are molecular keys that the body can automatically recognize and utilize. In other words, human-identical hormones are the perfect fit for a woman's genetic hormone receptor lock. When used for hormone replacement, human-identical hormones enter the bloodstream, attach to their appropriate receptor locks and safely and effectively reestablish optimum hormonal equilibrium. Human-identical hormones replace what is missing so that the female body has what it needs to feel and perform the way it was originally designed.

The Importance of Molecular-Identical Human Hormones

Naturally occurring hormones are created within your body. Human-identical hormones are made within a laboratory. They are made from scratch from hormone precursor molecules found in soybeans or wild yams. Human-identical hormones are identical to the ones your body naturally manufactures.

I would not be surprised if the idea of a laboratory makes you a bit uncomfortable, particularly after all the negative information I have shared with you about pharmaceutically manufactured synthetic HRTs. Let me explain the difference. In the process, I will also try to eliminate some of the confusion regarding terminology and establish a consistent vocabulary defining the different types of hormone therapies.

The terms "human-identical," "bio-identical," and "natural" are often used interchangeably to describe hormones that have a molecular structure that is natural to the human body. While "bio-identical" is a chemically correct term, I prefer to use the term "human-identical." It is a chemical term that is easier for most people to grasp. It says what it is.

I prefer not to use the term "natural" when discussing hormone replacement options. I find that too often patients confuse real hormones with herbal alternatives or botanical products, such as dietary soy, wild yam, or black cohosh. Also, many people think that Premarin is a "natural" hormone because it is composed of estrogen derived from the urine of horses. Again, while this equine hormone does occur within nature, it is not natural to the human body.

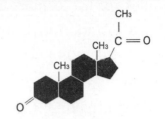

progesterone
Relative Binding Affinity = 100

Source: Human Pharmacology. Third Edition. (1998). Mosely.

The human body possesses progesterone receptors throughout almost all body tissues.

The progesterone produced by your ovaries fits perfectly into its receptor as nature intended and elicits the appropriate response.

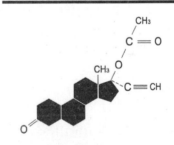

norethindrone acetate
Relative Binding Affinity = 6

Source: Human Pharmacology. Third Edition. (1998). Mosely.

The human body does not possess receptors for progestins (synthetic progesterone).

Synthetic molecules that are similar, but not the same molecular structure as progesterone produced in the human body <u>do not</u> fit perfectly into the body's receptor.

Progestin confuses the body's cells and receptor sites and stimulates a negative and defensive immune response.

As Dr. Joel Hargrove, a pioneer in the use of hormone therapies and the former Medical Director of the Menopause Center at Vanderbilt University, once said: "Premarin is a natural hormone only if your native food is hay." Just because a substance or molecular structure occurs within nature does not mean it is good for the human body. Think of hemlock. It occurs within nature but is very toxic to humans; no one would make the mistake of cooking and eating hemlock as they might spinach or turnip greens!

Again, the key to whether a hormone is human-identical is not where it is made but what its molecular structure looks like. A pharmacist or chemist has the ability to go into a lab, use plant extracts, and compound from scratch a hormone molecule that is an exact replica of the ones produced by the human endocrine system.

What about Other "Natural" Alternatives for HRT?

With continuing questions and rising concerns about synthetic HRT, many women have begun to experiment with "natural" alternatives. According to a 1997 study conducted by the North American Menopause Society, more than 30 percent of women who were suffering unpleasant symptoms associated with menopause tried herbal supplements or botanical products such as ginseng, black cohosh, dietary soy, fax seed, dong quai, evening primrose oil and wild yam.

Because my patients know that I am a believer in "natural" medicine, many of them ask me if they should try these botanical alternatives. I answer my patients with facts. To date, there is not enough strong evidence to support the efficacy of these remedies. In addition, while there are some anecdotal reports that these alternatives can impact hot flashes and night sweats, there is not sufficient clinical information to show any additional health benefits such as an impact on a woman's risk of cancer, osteoporosis or heart disease.

Biochemically, there is a reason these natural products don't work that well. The body is not set up to convert plant hormones into human-identical molecular structures from raw botanical materials. In other words, the human body does not have the ability to synthesize progesterone from wild yam or estrogen from soy. The hormones in these products are not in a form that is bioavailable; they are not in a form that can be readily absorbed and utilized by the human body at the cellular level.

When a woman uses a botanical product, such as wild yam cream, her body cannot absorb that product and transform its existing molecular structure into one that will fit the hormone receptor site. If the body can't recognize the molecular structure of these alternatives, it can't utilize them to restore hormonal balance and promote optimum health. While I applaud women for seeking safe and natural alternatives, it is sad and frustrating to witness them spending time and money to end up still suffering and feeling increasingly frustrated. While these "natural" alternatives may have some symptomatic value, I have found that only treatment with human-identical hormones can get these women the long-term relief and health results they both want and need.

Botanical: Soy

Theory: Contains isoflavones, which may mimic missing hormones enough to reduce hot flashes.

Findings: Italian researchers found that women who consumed 76 milligrams of isoflavones per day had 45% fewer hot flashes after three months; however, women given placebos had a 30% reduction; this suggests that the soy only had a modest effect.

Botanical: Black Cohosh

Theory: Some scientists believe this remedy may mimic the brain chemical serotonin, which perhaps weakens menopausal symptoms.

Findings: Several studies have found that this herb relieves hot flashes. But in a 2001 study at Columbia University, black cohosh was no better than placebos at reducing the number of hot flashes in breast-cancer survivors, though it may have made them less intense.

Botanical: Red Clover

Theory: Red clover is said to be one of nature's richest sources of isoflavones.

Findings: In one study, women who took 40 milligrams of red clover per day reduced hot flashes by 56%; however, the researchers didn't compare the results with the effect in women receiving no therapy.

Botanical: Evening-Primrose

Theory: It's not clear how evening-primrose oil stops hot flashes, though its potential anti-inflammatory qualities might help with other menopausal problems.

Findings: In a 1994 study, women who took four grams of evening-primrose oil each day for six months experienced a slight reduction in nighttime hot flashes. Primrose oil can also help with breast tenderness and bloating.

Botanical: Dong Quai

Theory: This Chinese herb is recommended for a variety of women's health problems.

Findings: It was once beleived to act like estrogen, but a 1997 study suggests otherwise. In that same 1997 study, women given a daily 4.5 gram dose of dong quai had 25% fewer hot flashes - the same effect as in women given placebos. While traditional healers prescribe dong quai in tandem with other herbs, products on the U.S. market do not.

Source: *Health.* January/February 2002

Why Haven't I Heard of Human-Identical Hormones Before?

If this is the first time you have heard or read anything about human-identical hormones, you are not alone. In fact, in 2003 the University of California in San Fransico's Women's Health Clinical Research Center released a study reporting that about a quarter of the women who stop taking synthetic HRT because of its risks wind up resuming the drug regimen because of menopause misery. According to Jan Herr of Kaiser Permanente of Northern California, many women are desperate for alternatives to relieve hot flashes and other menopausal symptoms. Some physicians are prescribing anti-depressants for symptomatic results, even if the patient is not depressed. It is a travesty that, despite the fact that there is sound scientific research and clinical data to support the safety and efficacy of human-identical hormones, this option for hormone replacement is still not widely acknowledged as a safe and effective alternative treatment.

Greed and ignorance are the primary reasons why human-identical hormones are not widely recognized and acknowledged as the treatment of choice for hormone imbalances. From a business perspective, there has been little financial incentive to fund medical education forums or launch a national public awareness campaign. Remember, whatever Power you believe designed the human body owns the chemical structure blueprint for human-identical hormones. This means that while human-identical hormones can be replicated in a laboratory, they cannot be patented by a pharmaceutical company. Without a patent, a pharmaceutical

"Synthetic hormones are made by altering the molecular structure of a hormone enough so that it can be patented. These maintain some of the activity of the natural hormone, but any change in the three-dimensional structure of a hormone, no matter how small, changes its biological effects on the cell in ways that are not completely understood. Frankly, I trust the wisdom coming from Mother Nature's millions of years of experimentation much more than I trust fifty years of bio-chemical wizardry from Father Pharmaceutical!"

Christiane Northrup, M.D.
Author of *The Wisdom of Menopause*

company cannot protect a product's competitive advantage and profit stream. There is nothing in it for them to help educate you - or your physician - on the health benefits of human-identical hormones.

The good news is that, as you read this, there is a groundswell of increasing awareness. As I indicated earlier, there have been several dedicated physicians, such as Joel Hargrove, Helene Leonetti, Jonathan Wright, David Zava, and the late John Lee, who have committed their work and their voices to educating women about both the dangers of synthetic HRT and the benefits of human-identical hormones. This pioneering group of doctors has risked the disdain of the traditional medical community by giving thousands of women a choice, and possibly saving their lives.

In the last few years, there have been more stirrings within the traditional medical community. The debacle of the WHI study has caused reputed medical research institutions to retract earlier endorsements of synthetic HRT and take another look at human-identical hormone therapy as an alternative. Such intensified focus has the potential to gain momentum and, eventually, translate through the medical schools and into the training and continuing education of practicing physicians.

While it is encouraging that the medical community is showing some signs of waking up, the fact that the media is beginning to educate the female consumer is even more exciting and will probably have the most dramatic impact in changing behaviors and prescribing patterns. In 2003, popular women's magazines like *"O" The Oprah Magazine, Good Housekeeping, More* and *Self* published articles warning of the dangers of synthetic hormone replacement and encouraging their readers to challenge their physicians regarding their choices for treating their symptoms of hormone imbalance.

Also in 2003, Dr. Phil and his wife Robin McGraw broadcast a national TV show entitled "Hormones From Hell." During their program, they interviewed women and a select group of medical experts to discuss the symptoms of hormone imbalance as well as several more natural alternatives to synthetic HRT, including human-identical hormone therapy. Dr. Phil and Robin had such an enthusiastic response from their viewers that they broadcast a sequel to "Hormones From Hell" just a few months later.

Many physicians might guffaw to think that their patients would trust medical information they get from the internet or watching TV talk shows more than they would the opinions of their own doctor. I don't think that any doctor should be so arrogant or naïve. In today's environment, the healthcare consumer is demanding information and making informed decisions, with or without his/her physician's participation or approval.

The output of the WHI study cost the medical community the faith of many women. Gone is the absolute trust that patients - and particularly women - once had for their physicians. As their frustration feeds their need to find an alternative, it can be expected that more and more women will learn about human-identical hormone therapy. If I were Dr. Phil and Robin, I would start my next sequel on hormone therapies. This one I would entitle: "Human-Identical Hormones: Hell Hath No Fury Like A Woman On Synthetic Hormones Who Was Not Told She Had A Better Choice!"

Why Use Human-Identical Hormones?

To Relieve Symptoms of Menopause Including:

- Hot Flashes and Night Sweats
- Increased Anxiety, Depression and Mood Swings
- Vaginal Dryness, Atrophy and Painful Urination
- Loss of Concentration and Memory
- Sleep Disturbances
- Diminished Sex Drive and Painful Intercourse
- Loss of Muscle Strength
- Urinary Incontinence

.... In Other Words,
TO GET YOUR LIFE BACK!

Chapter 5

Personalized Medicine: One Size Does Not Fit All

We have established that human-identical hormone replacement works within a woman's body to:

- Alleviate the symptoms caused by the body's natural decrease in production of hormones.

- Replace the hormones that have decreased in order to reestablish the body's optimum hormonal ratio.

- Bring the body back into hormonal balance.

- Catalyze the body's natural hormone receptor lock and key functions.

- Safely and effectively support/improve a woman's overall physical, mental, and emotional health.

If all the above is true - and it is - once a woman found out that human-identical hormone therapy existed and could improve both her health and the quality of her life, what woman wouldn't want to experience the benefits?

Every woman suffering from the symptoms of hormonal imbalance can potentially benefit from a regimen of human-identical hormones but <u>ONE SIZE DOES NOT FIT ALL</u>.

Estrogen Dominance: A Very Common and Extremely Dangerous Condition

Unfortunately, the majority of the medical community continues to regard the symptoms of hormone imbalance, and particularly menopause, as an estrogen deficiency disease. Consequently, when a woman with menopausal symptoms enters most physicians' offices, she will exit with a prescription for some form of estrogen replacement. If the estrogen is synthetic, you have learned that its molecular structure will be foreign to the body and, as a result, its biological effects will be unpredictable and even harmful. Still, even if the estrogen is human-identical, the addition of unopposed estrogen can be toxic.

Remember, every woman's body produces three sex hormones: estrogen, progesterone, and testosterone. As described in earlier chapters, hormonal production will decrease with age and the ratios of all three of these hormones will change over time. The rate of change will vary from woman to woman and will depend on both genetic and environmental factors. Production of progesterone is the first hormone to decline, then estrogen and, finally, testosterone.

In most women, hormonal ratios will begin to shift sometimes during the pre-menopausal years (e.g. a woman's thirties). Progesterone production begins to decrease while the body's production of estrogen and testosterone remains relatively stable. As a result, even at this early age, the ratio of estrogen to progesterone is upset, which fosters a biochemical situation of estrogen dominance within the body.

As stated in Chapter 1, for a healthy woman the rate of progesterone production drops approximately 120 times faster than estrogen production. This means that, no matter their age, most women suffering from the symptoms of hormone imbalance and/or menopause will be estrogen dominant. If a woman is overweight, her risk of being estrogen dominant is even greater. In addition to the human ovaries, the body's fatty tissues also make and store estrogen. Even after menopause, estrogen continues to be made in the body by a conversion of the adrenal steroid **androstenedione** found primarily in body fat.

If a high estrogen ratio remains unopposed and unbalanced, undesirable side effects will most certainly occur. The side effects resulting from estrogen dominance can be as irritating and uncomfortable as hot flashes, night sweats, headaches and weight gain or as debilitating and life threatening as breast or uterine cancer. Estrogen dominance can be a very dangerous condition.

Why is too much estrogen such a bad thing? The answer is derived from, first, examining the various types estrogens that the ovaries naturally produce and, then, coming to a deeper understanding of each of their respective roles. In Chapter 1, we briefly discussed the fact that "estrogen" is an umbrella term for a class of hormones responsible for female development through puberty and the menstrual cycle through the reproductive years. We then identified the three predominant natural estrogens as estrone (E1), estradiol (E2) and estriol (E3). The graph on the following page illustrates the relative amounts of each of these estrogens in a healthy premenopausal woman.

A woman's monthly hormonal interaction is extremely complex. In a nutshell, estrogen peaks in mid-cycle at the time of ovulation while progesterone begins to rise dramatically after ovulation, peaks and then quickly falls. If there is no pregnancy, the lining of the uterus (the endometrium) sloughs off through menstruation and then the next cycle begins.

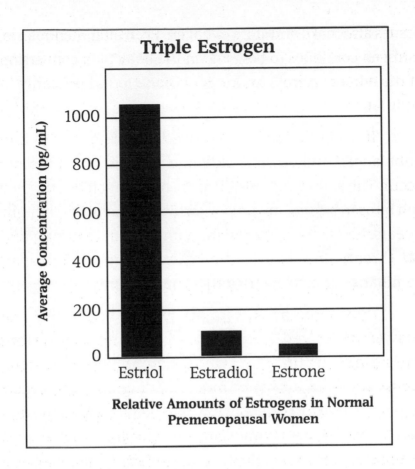

Triple Estrogen

Relative Amounts of Estrogens in Normal Premenopausal Women

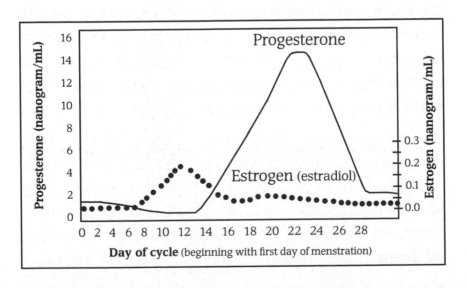

Estrone (E1) and estradiol (E2) both work within the body to increase expression of a gene (BCL-2) that causes cell division (development and growth), particularly in hormone-sensitive tissue such as the breast and uterine lining. If unchecked, this cell proliferation can lead to cancer. In fact, nearly every risk factor for breast and uterine cancer can be either directly or indirectly linked to an increase in estrone (E1), estradiol (E2) or their receptor activity. The close relationship between the risk of cancer and exposure to estrogen continues to be reviewed and validated.

Premarin, the synthetic HRT manufactured by Wyeth-Ayerst, is composed of 49.3% estrone (E1). This is almost ten times the ratio that occurs naturally within the body. Again, the potential consequences to women for whom this drug is prescribed should be of grave concern.

In contrast, estriol (E3) has been shown to have a protective effect against breast and uterine cancer. In 1994, Dr. Christiane Northrup's groundbreaking book *Women's Bodies, Women's Wisdom* highlighted estriol as an estrogen deserving more attention for its potential protective health benefits. She cited the outcomes of two clinical studies conducted by Dr. Henry Lemon over thirty years ago where estriol was shown to inhibit breast cancer development, first in mice and then in women with breast cancer. As a result of his findings, Dr. Lemon developed a formula called the "estrogen quotient" which reflected the ratio of the cancer-inhibiting estrogen (estriol/E3) to the cancer-promoting estrogens (estrone/E1 and estradiol/E2) in an individual woman.

Since Dr. Lemon's work, results of experiments in multiple laboratories over the last twenty years have continued to demonstrate that the body has a preferred ratio of "good" estrogens to "bad" estrogens. Research has shown that a large part of the cancer-inducing effect of estrogen involves the formation of agonistic metabolites of estrogen, especially 16-hydroxyestrone. Other metabolites, such as 2-hydroxyesterone and 2-hydoxyestradiol, offer protection against the potential carcinogenic effects of 16-alpha-hydroxyestrone.

How estrogen is metabolized in the body is determined by an individual's biochemical make-up, with some women producing more 2-hydroxy derivatives and others producing more 16-hydroxyesterone. The balance of anti- and pro-carcinogenic estrogen may be investigated with a urine test (trademarked Estronex) that measures the 2- and 16-hydroxyderivatives of estrone. If the 2/16 ratio is too low, the risk of cancer is greater.

Any woman with a family history, or who is simply concerned about her risk for breast or uterine cancer, could benefit from a urine test measuring her estrogen ratios. The motivation to take the test would surely be greater for a woman who has taken - or is taking - any form of supplemental estrogen. When the results from the urine test indicate a higher risk of cancer, there are actions that can be taken to turn the tide. Foods and supplements can be used to stimulate hepatic activity and increase the amount of favorable 2-hydroxy derivative within the body. For example, cruciferous vegetables such as broccoli and spinach have been shown to improve the production of "good" estrogen and foster an optimum 2/16 ratio. Also, improving omega-3 fatty acid intake can provide additional metabolic protection for estrogen metabolism.

I believe it is fair to say that most women over thirty-five are likely to be estrogen dominant. Are you? If you are, after what you have learned, why would you ever consider adding more estrogen into your system? What about the type of estrogen already in your body? Has your doctor ever recommended a urine test to determine your good/bad estrogen ratios? If you could, would you want to know if the type of estrogen in your body was putting you at greater risk to develop cancer? In my practice, I have found that most women with risk factors are willing to pee in a cup to find out.

Saliva Testing: A Personal Profile of Hormone Activity

A complete and individualized hormone profile is needed to provide a rational basis for correcting any hormone imbalance through diet, exercise, and/or human-identical hormone supplementation. While urine testing can give a reading of "good" estrogen levels versus "bad" estrogen levels, it does not provide an accurate reading of all the hormone activity within the body. In the last two chapters we have focused primarily on the hormones produced by the ovaries (e.g. estrogen, progesterone and testosterone). However, in Chapter 1 we also learned of the importance of the hormones secreted by the adrenal glands (e.g. epinephrine, DHEA and cortisol).

The interaction of estrogen, progesterone, testosterone and DHEA plays a vital role in maintaining the body's optimum functions. Because hormones produced by the adrenal glands play such a critical role in the body's response to stress and overexertion, it is also very important to measure their activity within the body. Consequently, knowledge of an imbalance in one or more of these hormones can illuminate the cause of health problems.

According to Dr. David Zava, Ph.D., a recognized expert on the biochemistry of human-identical hormones, saliva testing has been used in scientific testing for decades and has been shown to be a highly accurate tool for testing the spectrum of hormone activity and levels. The World Health Organization has used this method of hormone testing in worldwide comparisons of breast cancer among women living in industrialized versus non-industrialized countries. Many studies in the scientific literature have validated that saliva testing is the most reliable way to measure free, bioavailable hormone activity (the quantity of hormones actually doing their job in the body at the cellular level).

Most blood tests do not measure bioavailable hormone levels. When the endocrine system manufactures steroid hormones (e.g. estrogen, progesterone, testosterone), they are released into the bloodstream bound to carrier proteins. Only a small fraction (1-5%) of a given amount of a steroid hormone breaks loose from the carrier protein in the bloodstream and is free to enter the target tissues. This free or unbound hormone is what we want to measure, since it is active or bioavailable to act on the target tissues such as the breast, uterus, brain and skin.

Saliva collection is easy, can be done anywhere, any time and at a much lower cost. Blood serum testing is stressful, and the stress of a blood draw can sometimes alter the result. Blood has to be drawn at a doctor's office or drawing station, and it is more difficult to obtain samples at the desired times. Hormone concentration in blood serum can vary, depending on the time of day and month. This makes it especially difficult to schedule an optimum collection time. There is also an extra cost for drawing blood, independent of the cost for the test itself.

In contrast, hormone concentration in saliva is exceptionally stable, allowing wide latitude in collection and shipment. Samples can be stored at room temperature for at least a week without loss of activity, so samples can be shipped to the testing facility by regular mail. Blood, on the other hand, must be kept cool on ice packs, increasing the cost for shipping as well as the likelihood of error due to improper handling. Saliva tests are also less expensive than laboratory blood serum tests. A saliva hormone test does not require a prescription, except in the state of California. Because of their cost advantage and proven accuracy, most insurance carriers will now cover saliva hormone tests with a prescription from a physician.

As to the validity of saliva testing, the plethora of literature being published today strongly supports the thesis that saliva testing for all steroid hormones (estradiol, estriol, estrone, progesterone, testosterone, DHEA, cortisol) is as least as good as - and in many cases superior to - serum testing.

According to Dr. David Zava, "if a woman is taking hormones delivered topically through the skin in creams, gels, or patches, saliva testing more accurately reflects the body's uptake and response. In contrast, blood and urine assays significantly underestimate hormones delivered topically and often result in overdosing."

Why don't more physicians, and particularly gynecologists, make it standard practice to include a saliva test in their patients' annual exams? The answer is twofold. The first one you have heard before: ignorance. Most physicians are more familiar with blood serum numbers than they are with reading and interpreting hormone profile results from a saliva test.

Advantages of Saliva Hormone Testing

- Stress free
- Noninvasive (no needles)
- Less expensive & more convenient for both patients and physician
- Can be collected any time of the day/month, any place
- Does not require special processing prior to shipment (e.g. configuration, ice packs)
- Hormones remain stable in saliva for prolonged period of time
- Convenient shipping via U. S. mail
- More representative than blood serum of bioavailable steroid hormone levels

The second reason why saliva testing is not more common is that there are a limited number of laboratories capable of performing the tests. Laboratories performing saliva testing must have the technical expertise to either create their own tests or modify commercial test kits. Significant technical hurdles, beyond the technical expertise of most commercial testing laboratory personnel, must be overcome to make this transition.

> "As to convenience, accuracy, clinical relevance and cost, salivary testing is the far superior option."
> Dr. David Zava, Ph.D.

A saliva hormone test report will help a woman and her healthcare provider better understand how hormonal imbalances could be affecting her health and well-being. Most women will come to their doctor's offices seeking help because they are suffering from symptoms that are negatively impacting how they feel as well as the quality of their life. No woman is the same as another. Consequently, each woman will have her own unique profile including her individual medical history, age, menopausal status, menstrual cycle information and whether or not she has had her ovaries removed. Additional environmental factors such as personal or professional stresses all affect hormone levels and should be included on the test report.

If a woman is already taking any form of hormone therapy, the form and type of hormone therapy must be noted along with a description of the delivery mode (oral versus topical). The results of saliva testing should be integrated with an understanding of the patient's presenting symptoms in relationship to their hormone levels. Numerous studies and books have documented the correspondence between certain symptoms and the hormonal imbalances they evidence. Some of the most common symptoms that typically correspond to excesses and deficiencies of steroid hormones in women, are listed in the table below.

Indicate the symptoms you are experiencing as 0 (none), 1 (mild), 2 (moderate), 3 (severe).

⓪①②③ Hot Flashes	⓪①②③ Infertility Problems
⓪①②③ Goggy Thinking	⓪①②③ Nails Breaking or Brittle
⓪①②③ Heart Palpitations	⓪①②③ Rapid Heartbeat
⓪①②③ Aches & Pains	⓪①②③ Vaginal Dryness
⓪①②③ Allergies	⓪①②③ Tearful
⓪①②③ Sugar Cravings	⓪①②③ Sleep Disturbed
⓪①②③ Loss Scalp Hair	⓪①②③ Morning Fatigue
⓪①②③ Tender Breasts	⓪①②③ Stress
⓪①②③ Anxious	⓪①②③ Weight Gain - Waist
⓪①②③ Weight Gain - Hips	⓪①②③ Acne
⓪①②③ High Cholesterol	⓪①②③ Nervous
⓪①②② Hair Dry or Brittle	⓪①②③ Fibrocystic Breasts
⓪①②③ Constipation	⓪①②③ Decreased Muscle Size
⓪①②③ Hoarsness	⓪①②③ Slow Pulse Rate
⓪①②③ Night Sweats	⓪①②③ Thinning Skin
⓪①②③ Memory Laps	⓪①②③ Hearing Loss
⓪①②③ Bone Loss	⓪①②③ Incontinence
⓪①②③ Fibromyalgia	⓪①②③ Depressed
⓪①②③ Sensitivity To Chemicals	⓪①②③ Headaches
⓪①②③ Elevated Triglycerides	⓪①②③ Evening Fatigue
⓪①②③ Uterine Fibroids	⓪①②③ Cold Body Temperature
⓪①②③ Bleedling Changes	⓪①②③ Decreased Libido
⓪①②③ Water Retention	⓪①②③ Mood Swings
⓪①②③ Decreased Stamina	⓪①②③ Irritable
⓪①②③ Rapid Aging	⓪①②③ Goiter
⓪①②③ Deceased Sweating	⓪①②③ Other
⓪①②③ Increased Facial or Body Hair	⓪①②③ Swelling or Puffy Eyes, Face

Source: ZRT Laboratories, Beaverton, Oregon. CLIA Certified Laboratory

Ideally, a saliva hormone test should also help healthcare providers and their patients reach an educated decision about the right next steps, including options for human-identical hormone replacement.

Compounding Pharmacies: Formulating Personalized Prescriptions

Once a physician has a patient's individual hormone profile, he or she can prescribe a personalized formulation of human-identical hormones that can address the patient's individual needs. If each patient has their own unique hormonal profile, then it is not possible to manufacture a single pharmaceutical product that could meet the needs of each individual patient. This means that each patient will need to have a personalized prescription of human-identical hormones created - or compounded - just for them. This type of prescription is not readily filled at the local corner drug store, even if it is a national chain. This type of prescription will need to be prepared in a compounding pharmacy, which is certified and licensed to prepare prescriptions to order.

Compounding pharmacists can be a resource for those physicians who are interested in moving away from the use of synthetic HRT but do not have the experience or training to become skilled in new areas such as the use of saliva testing and the subsequent prescription of human-identical hormones. Today's compounding pharmacies can produce literally whatever the doctor orders, including various drug forms such as capsules, tablets, sublingual gels or creams.

Again, the physician and compounding pharmacist can work together to tailor the form of the drug so that it optimizes efficacy while also enhancing the patient's compliance.

If you've never heard of a compounding pharmacy before, here are some facts you might want to know:

- Every compounding pharmacy is licensed and inspected by the State Pharmacy Board.

- Compounding pharmacists are educated and trained to provide information regarding the formulation of human-identical hormones; they can reassure, educate, and provide physicians with safe dosage guidelines for human-identical hormone supplementation.

- All materials used in compounded formulations are subject to FDA inspection and the agency's Good Manufacturing Procedures code.

- The International Academy of Compounding Pharmacists (IACP) or the Professional Compounding Centers of America, Inc. (PCCA) are two excellent resources to help you - or your physician - locate a compounding pharmacy near you. Their 1-800 numbers, as well as their website addresses, are included in Chapter 14 "Resource Listing."

Many individuals become convinced of the benefits of human-identical hormones and then become frustrated because they have a hard time finding a physician who is knowledgeable enough about human-identical hormones to evaluate their personal hormone profile and get them what they want and need. This is, and will continue to be, a problem. Hopefully, this book will be one step taken to educate physicians and help rectify that situation.

In the meantime, I would advise against patients taking their treatment plans into their own hands. Many patients come to me after they have shopped the health food stores, or the Internet, and found some over-the-counter formulations of "natural" hormone therapies. While their intention to move away from synthetic formulations is one I support, I find that too many times these same patients spend a lot of money with little result.

There are several reasons why over-the-counter formulations are not as beneficial as compounded human-identical hormone therapies. First and foremost, a mass manufactured product can't possibly be expected to exactly match and replace the genetically determined hormonal balance of each individual. Secondly, not all over-the-counter formulations are the same: a layperson would have great difficulty reviewing the ingredient list and ensuring that they are getting the "right" ratio of the hormonal supplement that they desire. Finally, I support patients acting as informed consumers but I believe that the patient and physician should combine their knowledge and skill sets to come up with the best solution for each individual's situation. I continue to maintain that without a physician and an annual exam (that includes a pap smear, a mammogram and possibly a urine test measuring the anti- and pro-metabolites of estrogen) patients are in danger of just treating symptoms and, therein, missing the early signs of such life threatening diseases as breast or uterine cancer.

Over-the-counter formulations of human-identical hormone products probably won't hurt anyone, and they might actually help some. Still, what about those patients who could be helped more if they had a prescription compounded just for them based on their unique profile of hormonal imbalances? What about those patients who think that they are taking good care of themselves by steering away from synthetic HRT but who might be missing the signals that their body may be suffering from a disease that could require more intensive treatment than hormone replacement therapy?

In my practice, I have a compounding pharmacist onsite. I know that an effective and personalized treatment plan for my patients requires a clinical three-legged stool of expertise:

- My expertise as a physician and diagnostician;

- Each patient's personal "knowing" regarding her unique medical and family history, her presenting symptoms, and her current life situation; and

- The technical expertise of a compounding pharmacist to help me put in dosage form an individualized prescription of human-identical hormones

This approach to personalizing a human-identical hormone replacement program for each of my patients takes more time than if I could simply scratch off a prescription on a pad and have my patients run down to their corner drug store and get it filled with a mass-produced synthetic pharmaceutical product. Still, my time and extra effort is worth it. I see results every day that my patients report to me as "truly miraculous." As a physician who works with thousands of women suffering from hormonal imbalance every year, I am completely convinced that individualized prescriptions for human-identical hormone therapies are the safest and most effective treatment I can offer my patients. Even more, listening to each patient's story, evaluating her individual salivary hormone test, and integrating facts from her medical history has its return. In almost all cases, my patients exhibit a positive response only after a few weeks. When I prescribe human-identical hormone therapies for my patients, I am constantly reminded that one size will never fit all!

Chapter 6

Progesterone: The "Feel Good" Hormone

Progesterone Cream: Carol's "Gift From Heaven"

"Dr. Randolph, it is a MIRACLE! I actually feel good. I truly am beginning to like myself again. My family gratefully says that I am acting like my 'old self'. I have my life back and I can't thank you enough."

Even though I hear this refrain many times each week, I am always humbled by my patients' reaction to how they feel after being placed on a personalized regimen of human-identical hormones. This time the patient was Carol, the women whom I introduced as Case Study #1 in Chapter 2 (Carol/Heavy, Hot, and Angry at Forty-Seven Years Old). As you may recall, when I met Carol just a few months before, she had despairingly asked me to "just shoot her" if I couldn't treat and alleviate some of the menopausal symptoms she was suffering. Three months prior, at her initial visit, I had indicated to Carol that she was experiencing many of the unpleasant symptoms typically associated with perimenopause. I told her that these symptoms were the result of her aging body's decreased production of certain hormones. Then I helped Carol to understand that, without intervention, her hormonal imbalance would continue to negatively impact her body's physical, mental and emotional functions; however, I told her that I did have another option for her to consider.

Carol listened as I explained to her the opportunity to have replacement human-identical hormone therapy. I told her that, before I could begin to treat her, she would have to do a salivary test. Once I had her results in hand, I would be able to analyze her individual hormonal profile and determine what formulation of human-identical hormones would be required to re-establish her optimum hormonal equilibrium. Carol was skeptical, but also desperate for help. She agreed to move forward.

Below is an abbreviated version of Carol's salivary test results:

Hormone Tested	Within Normal Limits (WNL)	Deficiency (DEF)	Excess (EX)
Estrogen: -Estradiol -Estriol -Estrone	✔ ✔ ✔		
Progesterone		✔	
Testosterone	✔		
DHEA	✔		
Cortisol	✔		
Progesterone/ Estradiol (Pg/E2) Ratio*		✔	

*The Pg/E2 ratio is a key indicator of hormonal imbalance.

As I had suspected, not all of Carol's hormones were in balance. In examining Carol and reviewing her salivary test results, the most important finding was the deficiency in Carol's progesterone levels. Her body was not producing enough progesterone and, as a result, she was estrogen dominant. This deficiency was the primary underlying cause of the symptoms that had been driving Carol to the brink of despair: irritability, weight gain, hair loss, flaccid skin tone, hot flashes, and night sweats.

The fact that Carol was overweight was also an important contributing factor. There is a direct connection between body fat and estrogen. Increased body fat raises estrogen levels and estrogen dominance impacts the function of the thyroid in a manner that increases the body's tendency to accumulate even more body fat. I knew that Carol was caught in a negative cycle and would not begin to feel better until her hormones were back in balance. I would need to augment her body's production of progesterone. I was also certain that, once we began to resolve the fundamental issue of her estrogen dominance, we would begin to see a change in her weight.

I explained to Carol that, based on the findings of her tests, we needed to add more progesterone to her system. I expressed to her that I would like to prescribe human-identical progesterone in the form of a cream. The dosage would be 1/4teaspoon of cream applied twice daily. (Note: The advantages of a cream or transdermal delivery form will be addressed later in this chapter).

After answering Carol's questions, I gave her educational materials on human-identical hormones and an instruction chart on how to apply progesterone cream. After her individualized prescription was compounded in my pharmacy, I asked Carol to call me if she had any additional questions and I recommended that she schedule a three-month follow up consultation.

Now, three months later, Carol was in my office overflowing with reports of good results. "Dr. Randolph," she bubbled, "this progesterone cream has been a gift from heaven for me. My periods are regular again and the bleeding is back to what I would say is a normal monthly flow. I can sleep through the night without waking up in a dank sweat and feeling like I need to wring my pajamas out in the sink."

Carol went on, "I have lost 12 lbs and can fit into my skinny pants again. I'm not edgy and snapping at my family like I was before you put me on this cream. Dan, my husband, is so grateful that he sent you a bottle of champagne." At this Carol winked and handed me a bottle of Dom Perignon decorated with big red bow. Remembering that in her initial consultation Carol had reported a loss of sex drive, Dan's gift made me think that perhaps the human-identical hormone progesterone cream was also having some positive impact on Carol's libido. I repressed a smile as I accepted Dan's gift.

"Carol," I replied, "I am so glad that you feel better. Let's talk both about what happens now and what you can expect over time as you progress with your treatment regimen. Human-identical progesterone is all your body needs right now to reestablish your hormonal balance. However, hormonal balance and human-identical hormone replacement is not a one-time thing," I added. Over the next year or two your hormonal production will most likely continue to shift and your body's production of needed estrogen will decline. When you start to feel like your progesterone cream is no longer working effectively, you'll have a recurrence of some of your unpleasant symptoms; that is our signal for you to do another salivary test."

"Carol, I am glad we have your hormones back to where they need to be right now. I will continue to work with you over time to keep your hormones in balance so you can continue to feel like your 'old self' again."

Why Is Progesterone Such a "Wonder Hormone"?

When the production of progesterone is in optimum balance with the body's production of estrogen, progesterone demonstrates its benefits as a hormone. Progesterone is the hormone that is most crucial for:

- Survival of the ovum (egg) once fertilized (pregnancy)

- Protection against uterine cancer by preventing the overgrowth of the endometrium (lining of the uterus) that can be fueled by too much estrogen

- Protection against breast cancer and fibrocystic disease by preventing the proliferation of breast tissue cells that can be fueled by too much estrogen

- Protection against ovarian cancer by preventing the overgrowth of ovarian tissue cells that can be fueled by too much estrogen, and

- Stimulation of bone building that can prevent or treat osteoporosis.

In addition, progesterone counters the undesirable effects of estrogen dominance by:

- Serving as a natural anti-depressant

- Fostering a calming effect on the body

- Acting as a natural diuretic thereby preventing water retention or bloating

- Normalizing blood sugar levels

- Maintaining libido

- Promoting regular sleep patterns, and

- Restoring proper cell oxygen levels, thereby improving mental acuity and memory.

Let me offer a simple explanation of how progesterone plays other (non-reproductive) critical roles within the body. I hope you will forgive me because the metaphor I am going to use to explain this is a bit *male* but, then again, consider the source. Anyway, if I were a coach on a football team, progesterone would be my defense and estrogen my offense. When estrogen is unopposed (not blocked or balanced by progesterone) it wreaks havoc within the female body. Unopposed estrogen - or estrogen dominance - can cause a woman to suffer a gamut of symptoms from weight gain, mood swings, and memory loss to breast/uterine cancer, and heart disease.

Because the female body's production of progesterone is the first to decline, estrogen can begin to take over and run rampant with its ill effects long before a woman enters menopause. I have treated twenty- and thirty-year-old women who were estrogen dominant. These young women thought that they had decades to live before they would have to deal with symptoms of hormone imbalance. Before they were diagnosed, they thought hormone replacement was something for their mothers, not them.

 At whatever age estrogen dominance and its subsequent negative side effects begin, adding human-identical progesterone back into the system can be a proactive defense strategy. Again, like a football game that requires both an offense and defense to be on the field for the game to be played, *a healthy woman will need both estrogen and progesterone to be present and in balance.*

More About Progesterone

Progesterone is a 21-carbon hormone formed from steroid precursors in the ovary, testis, adrenal glands, placenta and glial cells in the central nervous system (CNS). It is present in highest concentration in the ovarian corpus luteum. Progesterone receptors are found in the uterus, CNS, mammary glands, pituitary, colon, lung and many other tissues. Synthesis of progesterone is stimulated by the luteinizing hormone (LH), which acts mainly to regulate the conversion of cholesterol to pregnelone, a progesterone precursor.

Role of Progesterone in Reproduction

LH stimulation of progesterone formation and release during the luteal phase occurs in anticipation of a fertilized egg. If a pregnancy does occur, the corpus luteum secretes the progesterone needed to maintain the pregnancy for about ten to twelve weeks, or until the placenta is large enough to take over. If the egg is not fertilized, progesterone release stops and the menstrual cycle begins again.

Sounds Good, but Can You Prove It? What the Research Shows

Medical literature provides clear physiological and biochemical evidence substantiating the many health benefits that result when the body's production of progesterone is normalized. For instance, Dr. Joel T. Hargrove, a clinical professor at Vanderbilt University Medical Center, frequently published multiple studies validating the efficacy (effectiveness) of human-identical progesterone replacement in many highly reputed medical journals.

The clinical trials conducted by Dr. Hargrove evidenced the critical role that progesterone plays in suppressing estrogen-dependent cell proliferation. Simply stated, cell proliferation (meaning overgrowth) can be a precursor for the development of cancerous tissue. Dr. Hargrove's work provided evidence that progesterone balances estrogen by turning off the cell growth mechanism. This means that progesterone can have a cancer-preventing effect within the body.

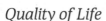

Quality of Life

Similar findings of progesterone improving overall quality of life have been reported by other nationally recognized centers of medical excellence. For instance, in the May 2000 issue of the *Journal of Women's Health*, the Mayo Clinic published a study reporting that women who included naturally-occurring (human-identical) progesterone in their hormone replacement regimen were more satisfied with their overall quality of life. Investigators followed 176 women whose prescribed hormone replacement therapy included human-identical progesterone with estrogen. They determined that, unlike synthetic progestin, human-identical progesterone did not negate the positive effect that estrogen can have on cholesterol levels.

Study participants also reported that they felt an improvement in several other health areas as a result of their progesterone therapy. According to Dr. Lorraine Fitzpatrick, a Mayo Clinic endocrinologist and the leading investigator of the study: "We already knew that progesterone can decrease some of the risks of estrogen replacement therapy such as increased risk of endometrial or uterine cancers. Now it seems that naturally-occurring (human-identical) progesterone can also reduce the occurrence of sleep disorders, hot flashes, anxiety, and symptoms of depression."

Cardiac Health

Progesterone is also good for heart health. Because heart disease is the number one killer of women in America, the effect of progesterone on cardiac health has also been an area of extensive research. You will recall that the Women's Health Initiative (WHI) trial indicated synthetic estrogen plus progestin (synthetic progesterone) increased cardiac risk. The good news is researchers have proven that for women on a hormonal replacement regimen that includes both estrogen and human-identical progesterone, progesterone actually serves to reduce coronary vascular activity. In other words, whether progesterone is produced within the body naturally or is a human-identical formulation added back into a woman's system, progesterone has definitively been shown to balance estrogen and have a cardio-protective effect.

The evidence that progesterone exerts a beneficial effect on cardiovascular function continues to accumulate:

- A recent study has shown that vaginally administered progesterone had a beneficial effect on cardiovascular health. Time to ischemia on a treadmill was increased in postmenopausal women who had cardiovascular disease. Source: Rosano GM, Webb CM, Chierchia S et al. (2000)

- Natural progesterone, but not medroxy progesterone acetate (synthetic progesterone), enhances the beneficial effect of estrogen on exercise-induced myocardial ischemia in postmenopausal women. Source: *Journal of American College of Cardiology* 36:2154-2159. (December 2000).

- In another recent study, Molinari indicated that an intraveneous infusion of progesterone increased blood flow in porcine mesenteric, iliac, and renal arteries via the release of nitrous oxide. Source: Molinari C, Battaglia A, Grossini E et al. (2001). "Effect of progesterone on peripheral blood flow in prepubertal female anesthetized pigs." *Journal of Vascular Research.* 38:569-577.

- With the use of cynomolgus monkeys, a study has shown that medroxyprogesterone acetate blunts the estradiol-induced release of nitrous oxide, a potent vasodilator. Source: Williams JK, Honore EK, Washburn SA et al. (1994). "Effects of hormone replacement therapy on reactivity of artherosclerotic coronary arteries in cynomolgus monkeys." *Journal of American College of Cardiology.* 224:1757-1761.

Breast Health

Breast cancer is the most frequently diagnosed cancer in women. Breast cancer is also hormone dependent. As has been previously described, estrogen increases proliferation of breast cells, and when uncontrolled, this cell proliferation results in cancer. Very simply, continuous exposure to high levels of unopposed estrogens will most definitely increase a woman's risk of getting breast cancer. The body has "too much estrogen" anytime the body's production of estrogen is not in equilibrium with its production of progesterone.

In contrast, progesterone functions within the body to inhibit cell proliferation. Studies in such highly respected clinical journals as *The Journal of the American Medical Association, Cancer Research, Lancet,* and *The New England Journal of Medicine* have validated the anti-carcinogenic properties of progesterone. Today the statistics are that one out of eight women in the United States will be diagnosed with breast cancer. Early detection of breast cancer is very important but prevention is a much more critical opportunity. The scientific study I would most like conducted is one that would show a reduction in the incidence of breast cancer because every woman in the United States had begun to augment her body's production of progesterone as soon as her hormone levels began to shift.

Osteoporosis

Bone density loss (osteoporosis) is another health concern for many women today. It is normal for bone tissue to break down and rebuild continuously, just like all the cells in our bodies. This process takes place when osteo**clast** cells dissolve old bone tissue (osteo**blast** cells stimulate new bone growth). Estrogen has a rate-limiting effect on osteoclasts: it only delays the breakdown of bone tissue. Human-identical progesterone, on the other hand, stimulates osteoblast cells (bone formation cells) that result in new bone growth.

Morris Noteloviz, M.D., Ph.D., states "Progesterone receptors are present in osteoblasts. Based on *in vivo* [in the body] and clinical studies, it is now believed that progesterone may stimulate new bone formation, although the mechanism has not yet been identified." Women using transdermal [transferred into the bloodstream through the skin] human-identical progesterone cream experienced an average of 7-8% bone mineral density increase in the first year, 4-5% in the second year, and 3-4% in the third year. Untreated women in this category typically lose 1.5% bone mineral density per year. With regard to the treatment and prevention of bone density loss, no other form of HRT or dietary supplementation has had as high a level of positive response as human-identical progesterone.

PMS

Have you or anyone you know ever suffered from PMS? Well, if so, here is news about progesterone that you will want to hear. In the early 1950s, a theory was advanced within medical communities that premenstrual syndrome (PMS) was caused by unopposed estrogen during the luteal phase of the menstrual cycle (the time between ovulation and the onset of the next mensus). To test this theory, researchers administered human-identical progesterone by intramuscular injection, vaginal or rectal suppository, or subcutaneous pellets. Progesterone resolved PMS symptoms in 83 percent of the women included in the study.

> "No, you are not losing your mind: you're just losing much-needed progesterone. When you don't have enough progesterone circulating, estrogen is the dominant hormone. Estrogen in overabundance makes you angry, edgy, short tempered, and anxious. At the same time, estrogen increases the water content of the cells in your brain making you groggy, fuzzy and unfocused."
>
> **Erika Schwartz, M.D.**, 2002, *The Hormone Solution.* pg 41.

Memory and Moods

How about memory and moods? Again, estrogen and progesterone need to be in balance for the brain to function as it should. Estrogen increases brain stimulation and fosters clear thinking and good memory. Progesterone is very important to the central nervous system. It has been proven to promote healthy sleep patterns and to promote a sense of calm. Progesterone is often referred to as the "feel good" hormone. While its effect on moods and a sense of well-being is very relevant, there is new evidence indicating that progesterone may play an even more critical role in long-term mental functioning. Recent research has suggested that an imbalance between estrogen and progesterone levels may be a precursor to Alzheimer's disease.

Weight Gain

Weight gain is another concern shared by many women as they age. The weight itself is only part of the problem, I am often told. Women complain to me about the change in the shape of their bodies, particularly the fact that fat seems to accumulate around their stomach, buttocks and thighs rather than being more evenly distributed over their entire body. Once again, progesterone can effectively address some of the biochemical reasons for this weight gain. Estrogen dominance causes an increase in thyroid binding globulin. When this occurs, the thyroid hormones are bound in such a way that the thyroid gland becomes dysfunctional. The degree of dysfunction is proportional to the degree of estrogen dominance. As we know from Chapter 1, the thyroid gland is best known for its metabolic function affecting weight. If the body does not have enough progesterone, women can diet and exercise with a vengeance and still not lose the weight they want. Progesterone is needed to equalize estrogen dominance and eliminate a hypothyroid condition so that, with a healthy diet and exercise, the body's metabolism will respond and weight loss can occur.

In addition, too much estrogen causes tissues around the abdominal area to retain water, or bloat. In younger women, this bloating is most noticeable around their menstrual cycle when their progesterone levels naturally drop to precipitate menstruation. As women age and their progesterone levels do not cycle back up during the month, then the resulting estrogen dominance causes the bloating to be a constant issue. This uncomfortable feeling is eliminated when progesterone balances the estrogen. Progesterone then acts as a natural diuretic, thereby reducing the bloating.

 Changes in blood sugar levels that occur with age and as a result of hormone imbalance are also linked to weight gain. As the body's production of progesterone decreases and circulating estrogen becomes dominant, insulin is released more rapidly and more often. When fluctuating hormones unnaturally stimulate insulin release, the body craves sugar. Food cravings can sometimes be uncontrollable. Many women report that they find themselves consuming many more sweets, even when they are not truly hungry. As a result, they ingest more calories than their bodies require. When progesterone is in balance with estrogen, it serves to temper insulin release, thereby normalizing blood sugar levels and reducing food cravings.

Sex Drive

Often overlooked or underplayed as a benefit of keeping your progesterone levels in balance is the link between a woman's progesterone levels and her sex drive. In his groundbreaking book, *What Your Doctor May Not Tell You About Menopause,* Dr. John R. Lee explains that he was intrigued about the underlying biochemical reason that so many women he treated as patients experienced a loss of sex drive with age. In his book, Dr. Lee indicates that his anecdotal findings prompted him to further investigation. When his patients took a saliva test, he found that their low libido frequently corresponded with a progesterone deficiency. Over the past decade, several studies have validated Dr. Lee's premise and confirmed a positive correlation between progesterone levels and sexual interest, desire, and response.

Progesterone: What I Believe to Be True

As a physician, I have prescribed human-identical progesterone for thousands of patients. Even after these many years, I never cease to be awed by my patients' response and gratitude. Once diagnosed and prescribed a compounded formulation of human-identical progesterone, most of my patients report a sense of well being that they had not experienced in years. Restful sleep, improved mood, sustained energy, weight loss, relief from hot flashes and restored libido are among human-identical progesterone's more immediate life-changing miracles.

I avidly review all the current research on hormone replacement options and am encouraged to find more and more studies validating the safety and efficacy of human-identical hormone replacement. Thankfully, however, in my own practice I am able to document progesterone's more long-term health benefits mostly by default. In other words, the fact that very few of my patients on human-identical progesterone also suffer from cancer, heart disease and/or osteoporosis is my real-life evidence. The more I prescribe and witness my patients' responses to human-identical progesterone, the more I am convinced that it is fair to regard progesterone as the body's "wonder hormone."

When is Over-The-Counter Progesterone Cream an Appropriate Treatment Option?

As a woman enters her mid-thirties and until she is in her late forties, she can be said to be pre-menopausal. A woman in this lifecycle is in her middle reproductive years. It is during these years that the balance of hormones produced by the endocrine system first begins to shift. As you have learned, progesterone, the "feel good" hormone, is the first hormone to decline and drops 120 times more rapidly than estrogen.

As progesterone begins to decline and estrogen becomes the dominant hormone within a woman's system, symptoms such as PMS, breast swelling, irregular periods, fluid retention, uterine fibroids, reduced libido and migraine headaches can occur. From their mid-thirties on, almost all women are estrogen dominant.

In many cases, this condition of estrogen dominance can be balanced by administering transdermal human-identical progesterone cream. Once the body's optimum hormonal ratio of estrogen to progesterone is restored, most unpleasant symptoms will be eliminated.

Human-identical progesterone can be dispensed in capsules, tablets, gelcaps, suppositories (vaginal or rectal), sublingual drops and creams. Topical creams have been shown to be the most effective mode of administration. When human-identical progesterone is applied topically, it is absorbed transdermally (through the skin) immediately into the bloodstream and then distributed and utilized in progesterone target tissues. Transdermally absorbed progesterone works within the body in essentially the same manner as the progesterone that is endogenously secreted (produced within the body) to enter the blood stream directly.

In contrast, oral routes of administration have been found to be much less effective. When progesterone comes into the body through the mouth it must go to the liver first to be metabolized, where some of the progesterone is lost in bile. What remains is then metabolized into more than thirty-five different biochemical substances before it can enter the bloodstream. Very simply, cream formulations of human-identical progesterone are much more effective than oral dosage forms. Transdermal absorption allows the body to receive, recognize and utilize human-identical progesterone in exactly the same manner it would the progesterone produced by the body's own ovaries. Biochemically speaking, you couldn't ask for anything better.

You can buy some form of "natural" progesterone cream over-the-counter in most health food stores. The good news is that it is available. The bad news is that you don't always know what you are getting. Most of the product labels do not specify whether or not they meet the following criteria for product excellence:

- Is the progesterone truly human-identical?

- Is the concentration appropriate for you?

- Do the hormones used in the formulation meet the United States Pharmacopoeia gold standards for quality and purity?

- Was the progesterone product actually compounded under the strict guidelines approved by the National Association of Compounding Pharmacists?

- Is the concentration of oil in the cream formulation one that will promote or inhibit transdermal absorption?

Because I never want to prescribe anything that I do not have the ultimate confidence in, I never recommended that my patients take a chance with any of these unknown and unproven progesterone products. When I first began to recommend human-identical progesterone cream, the only way I knew to assure that my patients actually got the product they needed was to make the progesterone cream myself. For several years, my compounding pharmacy literally formulated thousands of individual prescriptions.

I established a significant database of patients that I successfully treated with the human-identical hormone cream I personally prescribed and compounded. After some time, I recognized a pattern between the concentration of human-identical progesterone in the prescriptions I wrote and the positive response of my patients who used that formulation. Analysis of the correlation led me to standardize a transdermal formula for mass production.

My formula includes the concentrations of human-identical progesterone that I have found to be most effective. In addition, I worked with an FDA approved laboratory to develop a unique cream base that promotes maximum transdermal absorption and metabolism. The result is my own signature brand of over-the-counter progesterone cream: Dr. Randolph's Natural Progesterone Cream.

Most patients need to apply 1/4 to 1/2 teaspoon of my progesterone cream early morning and again in the evening before bedtime. The monthly schedule for application will vary according to a woman's presenting condition and whether or not she is still menstruating (see chart on pages 128-129). The good news about human-identical progesterone is that there are no known negative side effects. And with a cream formulation, if a woman is not getting the desired results with 1/4 teaspoon, she can safely increase her dosage by rubbing in just a bit more cream. The fact that a transdermal product form allows for a degree of self-monitoring and individual adjusting is another reason why I prefer creams to oral dosage forms. It is not as easy to modify your dosage and take just a "little bit more" of a pill or tablet.

Today, I provide a great deal of Dr. Randolph's Natural Progesterone Cream directly through my website: *www.safesthormones.com*. In addition, I am pleased to report that today there are several other over-the-counter progesterone creams that I have reviewed for quality and are assured that they too contain real progesterone. Among these are Emerita's Pro-Gest, Arbonne's PhytoProlief and Prolief Natural Balancing Creams, Products of Nature's Natural Woman progesterone cream, Life-flo Health Care Products' Progestacare, The Health and Science Research Institute's Serenity for Women progesterone cream, HM Enterprises' Happy PMS progesterone cream and Restored Balance, Inc.'s Restored Balance PMS/Menopausal progesterone cream. Again, if you have any doubt or concerns regarding any human-identical progesterone product, call the company and ask how many milligrams of progesterone per ounce the cream contains.

 While over-the-counter progesterone cream can help so many women, as a patient advocate I am adamant that this product is only one element in a comprehensive approach for hormone balancing and gynecological health. Any form of hormone replacement therapy should be monitored by a physician.

The following two pages contain information on how to use my natural progesterone cream.

Natural Progesterone Cream

1   Apply cream twice daily a.m. and p.m. to area marked number 1.

2   Continue rotating site of each cream application. After each morning and bedtime, move to the next numbered site (1, 2, 3, 4, 5, 6, 7, 8, 9).

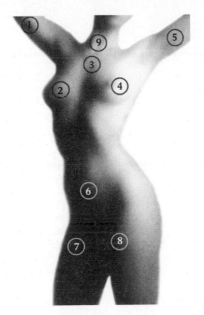

3   After you've reached site number 9 on the ninth day of cream application, start over with site number 1. Repeat rotation of cream application sites.

4   **CAUTION:** If you still have your uterus, do not take estrogen WITHOUT progesterone. This can cause precancerous cells to form in the uterine lining. **Taking Progesterone Alone Is Safe.**

SPECIAL INTRUCTIONS

PMS: Use 1/4 to 1/2 teaspoon twice a day from days 12-26 of your cycle.

Osteoporosis: Use 1/4 to 1/2 teaspoon twice a day for 25 days, take 5 days off. Repeat. After 3 months, decrease to 1/4 teaspoon twice a day. If using in conjunction with estrogen, apply cream everyday of month.

Endometriosis: Use 1/2 teaspoon twice a day from days 6 - 26 of your cycle.

Ovarian Cysts: 1/4 to 1/2 teaspoon twice a day from days 8 - 26 of your cycle.

Fibrocystic Breasts: Use 1/4 to 1/2 teaspoon twice a day from days 8 - 26 of your cycle.

Uterine Fibriods: Use 1/4 to 1/2 teaspoon twice a day from days 8-26 of your cycle.

Pre- or Peri-Menopause: Use 1/4 to 1/2 teaspoon twice a day from days 8-26 of your cycle. If using in conjunction with estrogen, apply cream every day of month.

Post-Menopause or Hysterectomy: Use 1/4 to 1/2 teaspoon twice a day for 25 days, take 5 days off. Repeat. After 3 months, decrease to 1/4 teaspoon twice a day. If using in conjunction with estrogen, apply cream every day of month.

Men: Use 1/4 to 1/2 teaspoon twice a day. Apply cream to same numbered sites as described on previous page.

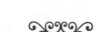

Chapter 7

Your Sex Hormones in Balance: A Healthy Ménage à Trois

In the last chapter, we discussed the pivotal role that progesterone plays within the body. As important as progesterone is, it is not a stand-alone hormone. Remember that the body produces three sex hormones: estrogen, progesterone and testosterone. All of these play a role in establishing hormonal equilibrium. Moreover, each hormone uniquely contributes to health and well-being.

In discussing hormonal balance, there are two key reasons that I chose to focus first on the critical importance of progesterone:

1. Progesterone production is the first to decline when the body's hormone production begins to shift. In most cases, the first time a woman begins to experience unpleasant symptoms associated with hormone imbalance, the symptoms occur because of the fact that her body is no longer producing enough progesterone.

2. When unpleasant symptoms associated with hormonal balance begin to occur, the medical community and the female consumer are still relatively uninformed when it comes to considering human-identical progesterone replacement as an initial treatment of choice.

Nevertheless, as the body ages, progesterone replacement alone will not be sufficient to keep the body's hormones in balance. As women go through "the change," the production of all their sex hormones - estrogen, progesterone and testosterone - will eventually diminish. Consequently, the challenge is to monitor the body's production of all three sex hormones and to know when and how to use human-identical hormone replacement therapies to bring the body back into equilibrium.

The *American Heritage Dictionary* defines a ménage à trois as a relationship in which three different individuals live and love in harmony together. The metaphor mirrors the relationship of the three sex hormones within the female body. In order for optimum health and wellbeing to occur, the body needs to have a supply of all three sex hormones: estrogen, progesterone, and testosterone. **Each hormone has a unique function within the body, but it is the interdependence of all three that defines hormone balance.** When estrogen, progesterone, and testosterone are present in the ratio that nature originally intended, the ménage à trois of the sex hormones supports physical and mental health as well as emotional harmony.

What Happens When All Three Sex Hormones Are Out of Balance?

Again, as a woman moves through menopause, the ovaries will gradually begin to decrease their production of all three sex hormones. Let's look back at Natalie (Case Study #2 from Chapter 2) for an example of what happens when this occurs.

As you may recall, Natalie was a fifty-three year old woman who could legitimately be classified as menopausal because she had not menstruated for two years. Natalie had come to see me after her previous physician diagnosed her with osteoporosis and recommended synthetic HRT as a treatment choice. Natalie had read enough to be confused and frightened by the idea of synthetic HRT. She had come to me to see if I might be able to recommend more natural and safe alternatives. Natalie had told me that she was a golfer who counted on her body to be strong and supportive. In addition to her concerns regarding bone density loss, Natalie had other unpleasant symptoms typically associated with progressive hormone imbalance: memory loss, urinary incontinence, abdominal bloating, insomnia, and a loss of libido.

As I do with the majority of my patients, I asked Natalie to do a salivary test so that I would have a clinical measurement of her body's hormone production. The table on the following page summarizes the results of her test.

With this kind of hormonal profile, I could certainly understand why Natalie had started our first conversation in tears when she reported that, "I must have Alzheimer's and everything else in my body is going wrong too." Natalie certainly wasn't one of those "crazy women going through 'the change.'" Biochemically and metabolically, her body was suffering from a severe deficit of all her sex hormones.

After menopause it is normal for the body's production of progesterone to fall to almost zero, while estrogen production initially decreases about 40-60 percent. Testosterone production does not decrease as rapidly as the others, but it is not unusual for post-menopausal women to also have a testosterone deficiency. In order to get Natalie's hormones back in balance, I would need to prescribe a comprehensive

Hormone Tested	Within Normal Limits (WNL)	Deficiency (DEF)	Excess (EX)
Estrogen: **-Estradiol**		✔	
-Estriol		✔	
-Estrone		✔	
Progesterone		✔	
Testosterone		✔	
DHEA	✔		
Cortisol	✔		
Progesterone/ Estradiol (Pg/E2) Ratio*		✔	

*The Pg/E2 ratio is a key indicator of hormonal imbalance.

human-identical hormone replacement regimen that incorporated the three natural estrogens, progesterone, and testosterone.

How Is Osteoporosis Linked with a Decline in Sex Hormones?

In addition to Natalie's hormonal profile, I was most concerned about the fact that her body was losing bone mass. Before coming to see me, Natalie's previous physician had measured her bone mass with a test called a DEXA (Dual-

Energy X-Ray Absorptionmetry) scan. This test is the latest in state-of-the-art technology; it uses two beams of x-rays to measure the bone mineral density (BMD) of hip, spine and entire body.

Bone Mass Density (BMD) status is usually considered in relative rather than absolute terms – as deviation from a reference standard rather than in grams per unit of volume. Two scores are in use. In other words, your diagnostic test data (Z-score) is compared to data from other healthy women within the same age group, race, etc. A BMD is abnormal if the test data is lower than the comparison group's (healthy women) range of test data. Again, the Z-score relates an individual's BMD to that of other individuals matched for age, sex and race.

In postmenopausal women, a negative Z-score of −2 or greater serves mainly to identify those needing evaluation for bone loss caused by something other than aging or menopause. Since osteoporosis bone loss is associated with aging and menopause, diagnosis of osteoporosis in post menopausal women requires use of the T-score, which relates their BMD to the mean of young adult pre-menopausal women. The more negative the number, expressed as SD (standard deviation), the greater the risk of fracture.

The table on the next page itemizes the current criteria for the densitometric diagnosis of osteoporosis, proposed by a study of the World Health Organization (WHO) in 1994 and now the international standard. The WHO definition of osteoporosis as T-score below −2.5 SD is an operational one, based on trial fracture data mostly from white postmenopausal women.

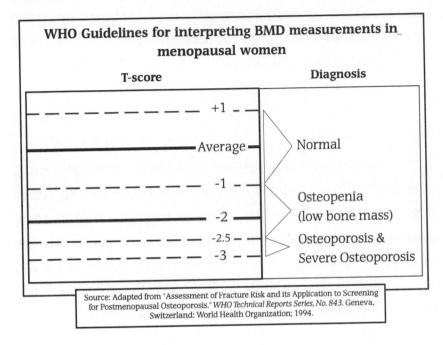

WHO Guidelines for interpreting BMD measurements in menopausal women

T-score	Diagnosis
+1	Normal
Average	
-1	Osteopenia (low bone mass)
-2	
-2.5	Osteoporosis &
-3	Severe Osteoporosis

Source: Adapted from "Assessment of Fracture Risk and its Application to Screening for Postmenopausal Osteoporosis." *WHO Technical Reports Series, No. 843.* Geneva, Switzerland: World Health Organization; 1994.

I reviewed Natalie's DEXA scan results: her BMD was more than 2.5 standard deviations below the average for her age, sex and race. I concurred with the diagnosis her previous physician had made: Natalie was definitely suffering from osteoporosis. When informed of her condition, Natalie became deeply distressed by the idea that her bones might be deteriorating and that, ultimately, her physical activities could be limited by this disease. According to the WHO, a BMD threshold of −2.5 is the best and most direct way to identify individuals most likely to have fractures in the future.

Many women share Natalie's fears regarding the negative impact that osteoporosis might have on quality of life. A progressive loss of bone mass and bone strength is one of the most common and disabling diseases affecting women in North America today. A conservative estimate is that more than 20 million women and 4 million men in the United States have osteoporosis. Osteoporosis is a major public health problem, as well as an individual one, with 1.5 million fractures occurring every year. The cost of hip fractures alone exceeds $14 billion annually. Worse, complications from a fractured hip are a frequent cause of death in older women.

Bone loss is not just an "old lady's disease" and it does not begin with menopause. In fact, bone mass typically begins to gradually decline when women are in their early thirties. As you may recall, a woman's estrogen levels are relatively stable during these years but progesterone levels are often less than optimal. This suggests a relationship between progesterone and the ability of bone tissues to renew and regenerate. During menopause, bone loss does tend to accelerate. This suggests a correlation between osteoporosis and a decline in the levels of all the sex hormones. In other words, the severity of osteoporosis increases as the body's hormonal imbalance becomes more and more extreme.

Despite the fact that women begin to exhibit bone density loss in their thirties - years before their estrogen levels begin to decline - mainstream medicine has focused on estrogen replacement as a panacea for treating osteoporosis. I find it deeply disappointing that many of my physician peers continue to suffer this kind of clinical tunnel vision. There are volumes of clinical studies supporting the reality that estrogen therapy alone is relatively ineffective for the restoration of bone mass. One of the most important factors is that estrogen dominance impedes the body's ability to absorb and utilize calcium.

Moreover, when estrogen replacement is unchecked by progesterone the body suffers unpleasant and some time dangerous side effects. Whether estrogen dominance occurs naturally as a result of hormonal shifts associated with age or whether the condition of estrogen dominance is fostered by unopposed estrogen replacement therapies, estrogen dominance has dire implications.

Sometimes patients suffering from osteoporosis will require that more than one hormone be replaced. Both estrogen and progesterone are needed to increase bone mass. Estrogen slows bone loss and progesterone stimulates new bone formation. As I first learned from Dr. John Lee, adding human-identical progesterone actively increases bone mass and density and, over time, can actually foster the reversal of osteoporosis. If estrogen levels have begun to decline, estrogen replacement may also be appropriate.

Testosterone also plays a role in bone building. Because, for most women, testosterone levels do not slough off until after menopause, testosterone therapy is not as immediately associated with osteoporosis. Research has shown, however, that the increase in bone density is twice a high in women supplemented with testosterone.

In Natalie's case, her testosterone levels were below normal limits, indicating to me that none of her sex hormones were in sufficient quantities to stimulate bone building. As I began to put together a comprehensive treatment plan for Natalie, the fact that she was suffering from osteoporosis only underscored her need for human-identical replacement of all her sex hormones.

What About Diet, Exercise, and Osteoporosis?

Hormone replacement is only one component in a comprehensive osteoporosis treatment plan. According to Dr. Norman Shealy, the founding president of the American Holistic Medical Association, calcium and magnesium supplementation are also key elements, as is exercise. Magnesium increases calcium absorption and also facilitates its role in bone formation.

The dietary answer is not simply "Drink More Milk." There is considerable controversy within the scientific community regarding the bio-availability of calcium in milk and milk products. The body requires magnesium to incorporate calcium into bone. Therein, an aggressive osteoporosis treatment plan should make dietary recommendations but, because the body may not be able to ingest and process enough of the right foods, I frequently recommend calcium, magnesium and other mineral supplements for my patients. I could see that in Natalie's case, she would benefit from some form of mineral supplementation.

I also was concerned about Natalie's diet for other reasons. When I inquired about her eating habits, Natalie had told me that she had been following a version of the Atkins Diet (a high protein/low carbohydrate meal regimen) for over a year. She reported that she had in fact lost weight and was mostly happy with the results.

I had a number of patients who all safely lost weight following a high protein/low carbohydrate diet; however, they were not suffering from bone density loss. Many clinical studies have proven that the body's absorption of calcium is decreased by high-meat protein and high-fat diets. The fact that Natalie was suffering from osteoporosis caused me to seriously question her choice of diets.

Finally, I examined Natalie's activity level. Physical activities, particularly weight bearing exercises, promote bone growth and renewal. Walking, biking, tennis, lifting weights and dancing are all good ways to promote bone health. Natalie indicated that golf was her primary mode of exercise. Unfortunately, Natalie always rode in a golf cart.

A Program to Balance Hormones and Build Bones

To effectively help Natalie, I needed to devise a personalized program to address both her hormone imbalance and her osteoporotic condition. Natalie's prescription for better health and stronger bones included hormone replacement, vitamins and mineral supplementation, and diet and exercise.

"Natalie's Prescription for Human-Identical Hormone Replacement"

Since Natalie's saliva test indicated that she was deficient in all three estrogens, I knew that we would need to replace all three in a way that would closely replicate the ratio of estrogen Natalie's body would have produced prior to menopause. With all this in mind, I prescribed for Natalie a human-identical estrogen formulation of 80% estriol, 15% estradiol and 5% estrone.

Human-Identical Estrogen/Triest: Triest is the name for the combination of all three estrogens (estrone/ E1, estradiol/E2, estriol/E3) often used in estrogen replacement therapy. Human-identical triple-estrogens are identical chemically and structurally to those produced within the body. They are synthesized from precursors found in wild yam or soy products. Since the raw materials cannot be recognized and used by the body's hormone receptor sites, special processing in a compounding pharmaceutical laboratory is required. As discussed in Chapter 5, the optimum ratio for the estrogens is:

- **estriol/E3**: approximately 60-80% of circulating estrogen

- **estradiol/E2**: approximately 10-20% of circulating estrogen

- **estrone/E1:** approximately 3-5% circulating estrogen

You may recall that during Natalie's initial consultation, she confided that her previous gynecologist had wanted to prescribe Premarin. Natalie had expressed concern regarding the potential negative side effects associated with synthetic estrogen therapy, and she had reason to be. Because Premarin is composed of approximately 49.3% of estrone, her body would have been supplemented with almost ten times the amount it normally would have produced.

Premarin also includes equilin, an additional hormone molecule that is made from horse urine. This issue was also addressed in Chapter 5 and the verdict on Premarin was not good. When foreign molecules enter the human system, side-effects can and should be expected. I was particularly glad that Natalie had taken control of her health and decided to come to see me to seek a safer and more natural alternative.

Finally, I had to determine what dosage form would work best for Natalie. Unlike progesterone, oral estrogen supplements are not as drastically metabolized in the liver. This means that human-identical estrogen can be dispensed in oral forms, such as capsules and tablets, or in topical forms such as gels and creams. I defer to patient preference and, in this case, Natalie chose to have her triest supplement in gel form. Her personalized prescription for estrogen gel was then made to order in my compounding pharmacy.

Human-Identical Progesterone: Given how low Natalie's progesterone levels were, I knew that progesterone replacement would be central to her treatment regimen. I recommended that she apply 1/4 to 1/2 teaspoon of Dr. Randolph's Natural Progesterone Cream twice a day. I instructed Natalie to begin with the 1/4 teaspoon dosage but, if she was not feeling some benefits after the first few days, to go ahead and increase to 1/2 teaspoon.

Human-Identical Testosterone: When given in pill form, testosterone is broken down by the liver and poorly absorbed. While testosterone gel works well for many people, I more frequently recommend sublingual testosterone drops because they are easily absorbed directly under the tongue into the blood stream. When I asked Natalie what form she would prefer, she indicated that the sublingual drops were fine. Her prescription for human-identical testosterone was then compounded in my pharmacy.

"Natalie's Prescription for Vitamin and Mineral Supplementation"

While I don't believe that dietary supplements should ever replace a good balanced diet, there are several "bone-building" natural substances that are safe and effective in the management of osteoporosis. For my patients with osteoporosis, I recommend that they supplement their daily dietary intake with 1500mg of absorbable calcium, 500 mg of magnesium, and a multi-vitamin that includes C, K, B6, B12, folic acid, and D3, as well as micronutrient metals such as zinc, copper, manganese, and boron.

I have my own brand of these vitamins and minerals and many of my patients prefer these, but I am aware that many other brands are readily available at most health food and drug stores. I always recommend that, when buying over-the-counter products, vitamins, and supplements, purchase a reputable brand, and also consult with your physician or pharmacist to ensure that the product contains a therapeutic dosage and doesn't include more fillers than substance.

Natalie was open to adding some vitamin and mineral therapy into her daily regimen if it could positively influence her bone structure. After our consultation, she went to the health food store to purchase the products I had recommended.

"Natalie's Prescription for Diet and Exercise"

I was concerned that Natalie's high protein diet could potentially sabotage her body's ability to absorb calcium, so I recommended that she stop using the Atkins Diet to plan her meals. We discussed the potential health benefits of adding some carbohydrates and more cruciferous vegetables - such as spinach, kale, cabbage and broccoli - back into her diet. Finally, I encouraged Natalie to consider managing her weight more by monitoring her caloric intake and moving more. We also discussed the importance of changing her physical activity to include more weight bearing exercise. As Dr. Stephen Holt

Natalie: Fifty-three year old woman.	
Presenting Concerns/Symptoms: Osteoporosis, Memory Loss, Urinary Incontinence, Abdominal Bloating, Insomnia, and Low Libido.	
TREATMENT PLAN	
Human-Identical Hormone Therapy	Triest Gel Progesterone Cream Testosterone Drops
Vitamins and Minerals	Calcium Magnesium Multi-Vitamin
Diet	Manage weight by monitoring caloric intake Move away from protein-only diet Increase intake of carbohydrates Increase intake of cruciferous vegetables
Exercise	Move more Walk the golf course Begin weight bearing exercises

said in his book *The Antiporosis Plan*, "without exercise there can be no bone health." I suggested to Natalie that perhaps she might consider walking versus riding a golf course when playing eighteen holes. She agreed to give it a try. She also said that there was a gym in her residential community that she had never even been inside. She said she might at least go in and "see what all those buff people do in there."

One Year Later: A Healthier, Happier, and Stronger Natalie (Case Study#2)

Natalie had come back to see me after six months and had had a good report. She told me that she was "religiously" following her treatment plan even though for the first several weeks she had to put post-it notes on her bathroom mirror to remind her to take all three of her human-identical hormone therapies as well as her daily regimen of vitamins and minerals. She also told me that she had started exercising more and, after a few blisters, had actually begun to enjoy walking eighteen holes when golfing. Natalie did tell me that she had stopped going to the gym because "all those women seem to dress up and put on mascara just to sweat it off." Instead she had bought some home video tapes instructing her on small weight lifting and she found that she liked to pop those in right before she watched the news in the evening.

I had asked Natalie to take another saliva test and, after I received the results, we had reviewed her human-identical hormone regimen. Because her progesterone levels were still not in what I considered optimum range, I instructed Natalie to use 1/4 teaspoon more per applications. We agreed that Natalie would "stay with her program" and come back for another consultation in six months.

When Natalie came back for her annual exam, she had another DEXA scan. After reviewing the results, she and I both were elated. Comparison of her pre- and post-treatment bone mineral density showed statistically significant increases in bone mass in her spine, neck and hip. Not only was Natalie's osteoporosis being held at bay, it was actually being reversed!

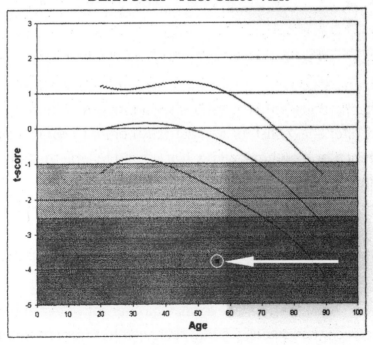

DEXA Scan - First Office Visit

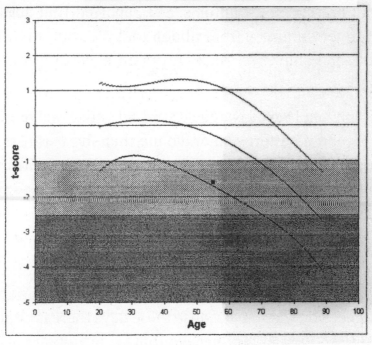

DEXA Scan - Annual Office Exam

Natalie had other good news. She had lost 10 lbs and all the exercise she was regularly doing had toned her muscles. According to Natalie, "I've never looked better in my golfing shorts."

She went on, "Dr. Randolph, remember that when I first came to see you I thought I was going crazy or had Alzheimer's? Well, I am here to tell you that I am thinking more clearly than I have in years. I no longer have to leave myself post-it notes on the bathroom mirror to tell me what I am supposed to do each day."

I was glad to hear that Natalie's human-identical hormone regimen seemed to be positively impacting her mental acuity. I looked at my notes from our previous consultations and asked her about any change in her other initial presenting symptoms. She reported that she was no longer suffering from abdominal bloating and, as a result, she didn't feel such an urgent need to urinate all day long.

When I asked Natalie if she had had any changes in her sleeping patterns, she told me that she was sleeping through the night. Remembering that on her first visit Natalie had told me that she and her dog Charmin stayed up all night watching movies, I laughingly asked her "How is Charmin adjusting to sleeping in the bed instead of on the sofa?"

Natalie also laughed when she told me, "Charmin still sleeps on the sofa because these days there is no room in my bed. Would you believe that - at my age - five months ago I met the nicest man on the golf course and we have hardly been out of each other's sight since? It is wonderful." I was glad to hear that Natalie was not only feeling better but that she had so many promising and joyful things happening in her life.

What she had just shared with me about her new relationship was a good segue for me to ask her about her previously low libido. Natalie assured me that she "felt like a woman again" and that, these days, "down there" (the term she used in our initial consultation) was working just fine.

Chapter 8
Hysterectomy Hysteria

Hysterectomy is a medical term commonly used both by physicians and the general public as an umbrella for several different types of surgical procedures. For instance:

- Technically, a *hysterectomy* is a surgical procedure that *only removes a woman's uterus and cervix but leaves the ovaries and fallopian tubes in place.* This procedure can be referred to as a <u>partial hysterectomy</u>;

- A <u>supra-cervical hysterectomy</u> is a partial hysterectomy that *removes the uterus but leaves the cervix, ovaries and fallopian tubes*;

- An <u>oophorectomy</u> is a surgical procedure that *removes an ovary*; this procedure can be unilateral (one ovary) or bi-lateral (both ovaries).

- A <u>bi-lateral salpingo-oophorectomy (BSO)</u> removes the both *ovaries and fallopian tubes.*

- When the uterus, tubes and ovaries are removed this procedure is referred to as a <u>complete hysterectomy</u>.

- A <u>total abdominal hysterectomy with BSO</u> removes the uterus, cervix, fallopian tubes and both ovaries. *This procedure is the most common type of hysterectomy performed on women in the United States.*

How Do I Know If a Hysterectomy Is the 'Right' Treatment Option for Me?

For decades, a large percentage of the gynecological physician community has promoted a complete surgical hysterectomy as the treatment of choice for women suffering from fibroid tumors, heavy uterine bleeding, pelvic discomfort, and/or endometriosis. The theory is: if they (your female organs) are bothering you, let's get rid of them, because once you have had children, you really don't need them any more. I find this theory flawed and the mode of thought behind it extremely short-sighted.

In her book *The Wisdom of Menopause*, Dr. Christiane Northrup addresses the fact that too many women have a hysterectomy unnecessarily and often for the wrong reasons. In the following passage from her book, Dr. Northrup openly challenges the practice patterns of many of our physician peers:

> *"Surgical removal of the uterus remains one of the most commonly performed operations in the United States - both doctors and their patients have been taught that these organs are dangerous at worst and expendable at best. One in three women in this country has had a hysterectomy by the age of sixty. And about 43 percent of women have their ovaries removed at the same time as their uterus, to prevent the possible development of ovarian cancer, despite the fact that the vast majority of women will never get ovarian cancer, but could definitely benefit from the hormones produced by our ovaries throughout the rest of our lives."*

A woman's female organs serve many purposes beyond reproduction. The ovaries play a crucial role in producing the sex hormones long after the reproductive years. The sex hormones produced by the ovaries (estrogen, progesterone and testosterone) play a role in maintaining a woman's health and vitality, as well as sex drive. Many physicians contend that it is better to do a *complete hysterectomy* removing all the female organs including the ovaries so as to eliminate a potential risk for ovarian cancer. There is substantial medical research illuminating how erroneous this thinking is.

Some women are appropriate candidates for a complete hysterectomy. There are risk factors, including genetics that can predispose a woman to be concerned about the likelihood of developing ovarian cancer. For these women, a complete hysterectomy may be the most appropriate and safe medical option. On the other hand, most women will never get ovarian cancer. For a high percentage of women, surgical removal of the ovaries is unnecessary.

In addition to the ovaries, keeping the uterus and cervix also serves a purpose. The uterus not only functions in the reproductive years to house a fetus: it also provides an ongoing source of blood supply to the ovaries through the uterine artery beyond the reproductive years. In a *partial hysterectomy*, the ovaries remain but both the uterus and cervix are removed. When the uterus is eliminated, the uterine artery is tied off and the blood flow to the ovaries is reduced. This can then reduce the ovaries' production of hormones. When the ovaries' hormonal production is prematurely reduced, it can cause a woman to enter menopause earlier than her biological clock might have dictated.

The uterus has another role within the body that should not be overlooked. It can help contribute or intensify a woman's sexual pleasure. During sexual intercourse, penetration can stimulate uterine contractions. The consequent rhythmic response has been found to contribute to an enhanced feeling of sexual pleasure. Many women report that after removal of their uterus, they experience less satisfying orgasms.

With a partial hysterectomy, the value of the cervix is also often undermined. Too frequently, surgeons tell their patients: "You are going to have to have surgery so you would be better off just getting it all cleaned out. Your cervix really doesn't play a critical role within the body anyway. You can easily live without it and, by taking it out, we also eliminate any later risk of cervical cancer." It makes me very sad when I learn that a woman has been convinced that this is true.

Every woman should have regular pap smears in order to proactively identify any pre-cancerous cells in the cervix. In a healthy woman, cervical cancer is not an imminent health threat. Moreover, the cervix plays several important roles within the body. First, the cervix is part of the normal pelvic floor and it helps to support the bladder. The nerves that go to the bladder run near the cervix. When these nerve pathways are cut, or disrupted, there is an impact on the bladder. Many women report that they suffer from increased urinary frequency and incontinence after a partial hysterectomy.

As with the uterus, the cervix also has a function in contributing to sexual pleasure. The nerves that run near the cervix also transverse the pelvis and the sides of the vagina. When the cervix is surgically removed, these nerve pathways are disrupted. This causes a lessening of sensation in the vaginal area. Furthermore, some men confide that during intercourse, they enjoy the sensation when the head of their penis brushes the cervix, or ceiling of the vagina. When the cervix is removed, the vagina becomes a kind of closed pouch.

I believe that every gynecologist should make it their standard protocol to attempt to intervene medically before reaching for a knife. In my own practice I have many women who suffer from the conditions previously described; however, I try treating them first with non-invasive measures including human-identical hormone therapy. Often I find that these non-surgical interventions prove successful in shrinking fibroid tumors, reducing uterine bleeding, and improving pelvic pain. Surgical intervention is always my last resort.

On the other hand, as a physician who treats thousands of women who have had a hysterectomy and as a surgeon who continues to perform hysterectomies, let me underscore that there are most definitely times when some type of surgical intervention is needed. I, myself, am a gynecological surgeon and I have patients whose presenting symptoms (fibroids, intractable bleeding, endometriosis, unrelenting pelvic pain) do not respond to non-invasive medical intervention. I have other patients who just want to "get on with it" and make surgical intervention their first round treatment choice. In these cases, I perform a hysterectomy and acknowledge that the procedure can provide relief and be a blessing for many women.

When appropriate, I prefer to perform a *supra-cervical hysterectomy*. This procedure removes the uterus but leaves the ovaries, fallopian tubes and cervix. If, in the future, pap smears indicate pre-cancer cells or cancer cells in the cervix, or if cancer is suspected in any of the other female organs, these issues can be addressed and the organ in question removed without another invasive surgical process requiring an incision. The procedure would be performed laproscopically through small abdominal incisions, or the cervix can be removed through the vagina.

My purpose in sharing with you all of this information is to educate, enlighten, and open your mind to options. Hopefully you are now aware that a hysterectomy is not a necessary rite of passage into or through your mid-life years. No one - including your doctor - can decide for you how to care for your health and your body.

If you have been suffering from one or more of the previously described symptoms, your doctor may be recommending that you have a hysterectomy. Your doctor may or may not be right. You will always have the final say as to whether a hysterectomy is the 'right' treatment option for you.

How Hormone Production Changes after Hysterectomy

Obviously a hysterectomy eliminates a woman's capacity to reproduce and her body will no longer be able to produce the sex hormones it needs to support optimum health and quality of life. This key issue must be recognized and addressed when a woman has a complete hysterectomy.

Women who have a complete hysterectomy (removal of the uterus, fallopian tubes, and ovaries) will immediately be thrust into menopause. In these cases, the onset of menopause has absolutely no correlation to a woman's age or lifecycle. Surgery will have removed the female body's capacity to produce any of the sex hormones. When this occurs, we say that a woman has entered artificial - or surgical - menopause. It can be expected that the body will go into a kind of shock. The resulting physical, mental, and emotional effects can be quite severe and even debilitating without an aggressive and comprehensive program for hormone replacement.

Even a partial hysterectomy that leaves the ovaries in place can affect hormone production. When surgery results in a permanent disruption of the blood flow to the ovaries, hormone production can decrease. It can be expected that a condition of estrogen dominance will be accelerated and will most likely foster the advent of many uncomfortable side effects most often associated with peri-menopause and menopause: hot flashes, night sweats, memory loss, low libido, thinned vaginal walls, fatigue, and mood swings. The medical fact is that a partial hysterectomy can catalyze premature menopause for most women. Again, hormone replacement will be required to address the cause and symptoms of the body's sudden imbalance of hormone production.

Too many women under the age of forty enter artificial menopause as a result of some form of medical intervention. In addition to surgery, other causes of artificial menopause include chemotherapy or radiation of the pelvic region. There is a body of scientific evidence suggesting that women who undergo premature menopause are more likely to develop some form of dementia. Dementia is more extreme than the fuzzy-thinking that is a common complaint of women in natural menopause. I believe that the cause of this dementia can be tied back to the rapid acceleration of estrogen dominance, which is supported by recent clinical studies linking synthetic HRT, and particularly synthetic estrogen, to Alzheimer's disease.

Can Human-Identical Hormones Help Me Feel Like a Woman Again?

I hear this question all the time. I must admit that every time a woman tells me that a surgical procedure has affected her sense of self-esteem, my heart breaks. I am so aware that every woman is much more than the sum of her pelvic organs. When a woman's hormones are out of balance, she just feels bad inside and out and can have trouble staying in touch with the essence of her feminine self.

Addressing the physical issue at hand is the first step in helping women who have had a hysterectomy to begin to feel like themselves again. Again, surgery has essentially slam-dunked these women into artificial menopause. Unlike natural menopause where the body's production of the sex hormones changes gradually and the body has time to adjust, women who have had a hysterectomy have little time to prepare for the gamut of symptoms their body/mind/emotions may evidence post-surgery. It is no wonder that, after a hysterectomy, many women despair and wonder if they have lost the spirit of their womanhood.

Most unenlightened gynecologists recommend only estrogen therapy after a complete hysterectomy. This is a very ill-advised approach. When a woman's body has had a surgery that eliminates the production of all her sex hormones, replacing estrogen alone can do more harm than good. Women on an estrogen-only therapeutic regimen will be medically thrust into an estrogen dominant condition and it can be expected that they will very quickly become symptomatic.

Physicians who attempt to help their patients with HRT must recognize two things:

1. The need to replace what is missing. A woman who has had a complete hysterectomy will require estrogen, progesterone and testosterone to restore her hormonal balance.

2. The principal of HRT can backfire and cause extremely negative side effects if the physician prescribes synthetic rather than human-identical HRT.

Human-identical hormone therapy must be recognized as the treatment of choice. It is essential to move forward with an aggressive regimen of human-identical hormone formulations for all three sex hormones (estrogen, progesterone and testosterone). For women who are going through menopause naturally, or for those who have had surgery but still have at least one of their ovaries in place, a salivary test is the first step in getting a baseline reading before developing a personalized regimen for hormone replacement.

For women who have had a complete hysterectomy, however, I already know that all their sex hormone levels will be deficient. For these women, I immediately start them on a comprehensive human-identical hormone replacement regimen and then have them do a salivary test in six to eight weeks so that I can see how they are doing, and adjust their dosages or regimen as needed.

Human-identical hormone replacement is just as important after a partial hysterectomy. A few years back I consulted with a very informed forty-two year old woman, Nancy. She had a partial hysterectomy at thirty-eight years of age after being diagnosed with fibroid tumors. Prior to the surgery, she knew that only one of her ovaries was cystic. Despite the advice of her previous physician who wanted to perform a complete hysterectomy, Nancy had researched her options and determined that she wanted a partial hysterectomy that left the healthy ovary in place.

When she came to see me, four years after her surgery, Nancy was disappointed that she was beginning to suffer many symptoms that signaled her body was moving into menopause. "Dr. Randolph," she told me, "I thought that if I kept one ovary it might be possible that it would be ten to twelve more years before I would go through 'the change.' I feel like my body and mind are drying up on me. Sex is painful."

Nancy continued, "I know this sounds silly, but I just don't feel pretty any more. I look in the mirror and I look like my mother did when she was in her mid-fifties and had been going through menopause for several years. Please help me; I don't want to turn into an old crone while I am still this young. I thought that if I kept my ovary this wouldn't happen to me now. What is going on?"

I explained to Nancy that she was suffering from the

symptoms of premature menopause. I concurred with her past decision to keep her ovary. She had most certainly delayed the onset of premature menopause, but because the blood supply to her remaining ovary had been disrupted and one ovary does not always have the capacity to do the work of two ovaries, it was likely that she would enter menopause sooner than if she had not had surgery. It was also obvious that Nancy's symptoms were indicative of a pretty extreme hormonal imbalance, but before I could treat her, we needed to know to what degree.

I asked Nancy do a salivary test to get her baseline. The following table highlights her results:

Hormone Tested	Within Normal Limits (WNL)	Deficiency (DEF)	Excess (EX)
Estrogen: -Estradiol		✔	
-Estriol		✔	
-Estrone		✔	
Progesterone		✔	
Testosterone		✔	
DHEA	✔		
Cortisol	✔		
Progesterone/ Estradiol (Pg/E2) Ratio*		✔	

*The Pg/E2 ratio is a key indicator of hormonal imbalance.

Forty-two or not, Nancy was showing all the signs of a menopausal woman. Her laboratory report verified that she was. Her serum FSH (follicle stimulating hormone level) was 48; a level of 30 or greater indicates that a woman has entered menopause. No wonder she reported that she felt and looked like her mother at fifty-five. I started her on comprehensive regimen of human-identical estrogen (Triest), progesterone cream, and sublingual testosterone drops. We scheduled a three-month follow-up appointment but only three weeks later Nancy called me to report, "My hot flashes are 100 percent gone. I can't believe it. Also, I am not experiencing the painful vaginal dryness that I have been suffering from for over a year. I am starting to feel like a woman again. How is this possible?"

I explained to Nancy that the human-identical hormonal program of estrogen, progesterone, and testosterone she was taking was most likely responsible for alleviating her symptoms. Also, I told her that many women on progesterone cream reported a decrease in vaginal dryness after only a few weeks. I hung up feeling glad that it seemed the human-identical hormones were having a positive effect for Nancy so soon, and that perhaps over the next few months she would have more evidence that she was still very much a woman and her feared transformation into a wise old crone was still far into her future.

What Happened to Barbara and Bob (Case Study #3)

For another example of the impact of hysterectomy and consequent surgical or artificial menopause, let's look back to Chapter 2 and Case Study #3: Barbara and Bob. As you may recall, Barbara had had a complete hysterectomy at forty-one years of age. Bob had contacted me two years after Barbara's surgery because he was worried that she seemed to be severely depressed. Moreover, Bob had confided that Barbara's breasts were "really lumpy" and that she had little or no interest in sex. Finally, Bob had wondered if the synthetic estrogen Barbara's doctor had placed her on was really "safe."

I had instructed Bob to share one of my videos on human-identical hormones with Barbara and, if she was interested after viewing it, to have her call my office to schedule a consultation. Barbara called within a week and was in my office just a few weeks later. She repeated what Bob had told me: she was very depressed, constantly fatigued and had little or no interest in sex. I examined her and validated that her breasts were fibrocystic, or "lumpy," as Bob had said.

One thing that Bob had forgotten to mention was that, at 5'4" and 197 lbs, Barbara was extremely overweight. Barbara said that she had always been "stocky" but since her hysterectomy, she had put on about thirty or forty pounds. I knew that Barbara's obesity was a major health concern and that it was probably contributing to the extremes of her menopausal symptoms. I was also concerned about the relationship between Barbara's weight and her breast health. Let's see why.

As with all my patients concerned about hormonal issues, Barbara did a saliva test. I also ordered a mammogram and a urinary test to assess the ratio of urinary hydroxylated estrogen metabolites. The results of Barbara's saliva test were:

Hormone Tested	Within Normal Limits (WNL)	Deficiency (DEF)	Excess (EX)
Estrogen: -Estradiol			✔
-Estriol	✔		
-Estrone			✔
Progesterone		✔	
Testosterone		✔	
DHEA	✔		
Cortisol	✔		
Progesterone/ Estradiol (Pg/E2) Ratio*		✔	

*The Pg/E2 ratio is a key indicator of hormonal imbalance.

Barbara was very obviously suffering from estrogen dominance. Of great concern to me was that it was her estrone (E1) and estradiol (E2) levels that were in excess while her estriol (E3) levels were within normal limits. As we discussed in Chapter 5, estrone (E1) and estradiol (E2) work within the body to cause cell division and growth while estriol (E3) has been shown to have a protective effect against cell proliferation in the breast and uterine tissues. These results were not surprising to me but the evidence of excess in the cancer promoting estrogens did validate my concerns.

You may be wondering: "If Barbara had a hysterectomy, where was all that estrogen in her body coming from?" First, remember that Barbara's previous physician had her taking Premarin. Her synthetic HRT was partially responsible for raising Barbara's estrogen levels, but her weight was also a contributing factor.

As we have discussed in earlier chapters, the ovaries do not only produce estrogen: body fat also raises estrogen levels. For years, the medical community has recognized the connection between fat and estrogen: more fat = more estrogen. Also, the American Cancer Society has established that breast cancer is strongly dependent on body weight.

Barbara's mammogram verified that her breasts were fibrocystic but showed no indication of cancerous tumors. This was very good news. Barbara's urinary test, however, indicated a very low 2/16 hydrox-estrogen ratio. A low 2/16 ratio corresponds to an increased risk of estrogen-dependent tumors.

Barbara was certainly caught in a dangerously negative and toxic cycle. Her hysterectomy had fostered hormone issues that were now contributing to her weight gain and depression. Barbara immediately agreed to switch from Premarin to human-identical HRT after I explained to her the many health issues associated with synthetic HRT. Still, she and I both knew we had to address her other health concerns. Her weight gain and hormone issues were increasing her risk for breast cancer. All were negatively impacting her emotional health.

I knew that I had to address how both Barbara's hysterectomy and her weight were impacting her hormonal functioning before we could improve her physical, mental, and emotional health. Human-identical hormone therapy was the first step in giving her some relief but it was only one part of a plan to improve her health and sense of well-being. Barbara needed a "whole woman" approach. I wanted to begin an aggressive and proactive plan to reduce Barbara's weight and therein decrease her risk for breast cancer. Her saliva test results helped me map a personalized treatment plan for Barbara.

"Barbara's Prescription for Human-Identical Hormone Therapy"

Progesterone cream to balance the effects of excess estrogen was the pivot of the plan. Testosterone therapy was also part of the regimen. Barbara's hormone issues were contributing to her depression, her loss of libido, her fibrocystic breasts and her weight gain.

"Barbara's Prescription for Vitamins and Supplements"

I recommended that Barbara take a good multi-vitamin. In addition, I asked her to start taking the following supplements:

- D.I.M. (Diindolymethane) (100 mg twice a day): this supplement has been clinically proven to improve the body's estrogen metabolism by converting "bad"

estrogen to "good" estrogen, and

• Calcium-D-Glucarate (500 mg twice a day): this supplement causes excess estrogen to be excreted from the body through the colon.

"Barbara's Prescription for Diet and Exercise"

Barbara had to learn how to eat to lose weight. In addition to counting calories, Barbara agreed to see a nutritionist I recommended. The nutritionist and I conferred and then agreed that Barbara's meal plan should be dense with cruciferous vegetables like broccoli. Studies have shown that these vegetables nutritionally increase the low 2/16 hydroxy-estrogen ratio. In addition, I recommended flaxseed oil capsules as a supplement because they too have been found to improve the 2/16 hydroxy-estrogen ratios. In addition to dietary recommendations, the nutritionist also suggested that Barbara reduce her intake of caffeine, which has also been tied to fibrocystic disease.

Because of her weight, I knew that Barbara would need an exercise plan that wouldn't put too much stress on her joints. We talked about options and Barbara said that she had always liked to swim but was now too embarrassed to get into a swimsuit. I told Barbara about a water aerobics class that I knew of where pretty much everybody who went was quite overweight, so there was no possibility of being ridiculed. Barbara agreed to check it out.

"Barbara's Prescription for Mind/Body Awareness"

I was very concerned about Barbara's depression and wondered out loud to her if it might be beneficial for her to see a psychologist or psychiatrist while we were addressing the underlying issue of her hormone imbalance. She flatly refused. Finally, I suggested that Barbara might consider reading some books or connecting with some groups engaged in some forms of mind/body techniques such as yoga, meditation and/or visualization. I shared with her that many of my patients reported to me that, before they could see the changes in their bodies, they "saw" them in their mind. She said "didn't like all that new-agey stuff" stuff but that she would look into it. "Anything to help. Maybe I will get Bob to go with me."

Three months later Barbara and Bob were both in my office. Barbara told me that her moods were much better and that she no longer spent her evenings on the sofa crying. She had lost 20 lbs. and was still losing weight. She was taking her supplements every day and saw the nutritionist once a month to tweak her diet and menu plans.

Barbara told me that she "loved the water aerobics" and had also taken up dancing. Bob had suggested that they take ballroom dancing lessons together and they loved it. Now they were considering a salsa class. I asked Barbara about her sex drive and she took Bob's hand and told me "I want to have sex with my husband again, Dr. Randolph. That part is wonderful but intercourse is still a little painful." We discussed lubricants and vaginal estriol cream.

Barbara had gone to one yoga class and hated it: "too many skinny people in tights!" She had, however, listened to a couple of audiotapes on visualization and found those quite inspiring. "Every time I start to think of myself as fat, old, and ugly, I get quiet for a minute. I then picture my grandmother as she was in her eighties: cameo-like skin, a still strong and lithe body, and a radiant smile. I hold that picture in my mind until I could put my face where hers was. I think that maybe I am programming my cells to believe that is who I am growing into."

When I first met her, Barbara's hysterectomy and subsequent estrogen dominance was fostering physical, mental and emotional chaos in her body. With so many positive things going on, I anticipated that a follow-up saliva test would substantiate that Barbara's hormones were now more in balance.

I was right. Barbara's second saliva test validated that we were on the right track: she was no longer estrogen dominant. Her urinary test showed that her 2/16 hydroxy-estrogen ratios had improved, but it was still too low. I told Barbara that I wanted to make sure we kept a close watch on this. I asked her to come back in another three months to repeat the test. Also, she was to not to miss her yearly mammogram or Pap smear. I remained highly vigilant regarding Barbara's risk for breast cancer.

Before they left the consultation room to schedule Barbara's next three-month follow-up consultation, Bob shook my hand. "Dr. Randolph," he said, "I thought that I had lost my wife forever. When Barbara had that hysterectomy it was as if that doctor had somehow surgically removed the soul of the woman I married. When I called you six months ago, I was desperate. Now, Barbara's health is improving and so is the health of our marriage. In fact, I don't think I have ever been more in love with my wife than I am today."

He continued, "You may think this is really strange, Dr. Randolph, but - while I would never want Barbara to have to have surgery again - in a weird way I think that Barbara's hysterectomy has turned out to be a kind of irregular blessing. Barbara tells me that she feels more empowered to take care of her health and her weight. I am so very grateful that you educated us both about the dangers of synthetic HRT, and particularly that drug Premarin that Barbara's old doctor had her on. Now, I am relieved that you have her risk for breast cancer high on the radar screen. Most of all, Dr. Randolph, this human-identical hormone therapy that you put her on seems to literally be a godsend. Thank you."

As I walked out of that consultation room I wished that I could share Barbara and Bob's story with my physician peers who do hysterectomies every day and never think to consider human-identical hormone therapy as an essential component of a post-surgical plan. This chapter brings that wish to life.

Chapter 9
Adrenal Exhaustion: Stress, Fatigue, and Accelerated Aging

Fatigue is a common health complaint but one that is too often dismissed by the individual or not given enough credence by the medical community. Our modern world moves so fast that most people today seem to accept being constantly tired as a normal state of being. It is not. In my practice, I recognize that a patient's complaint of constant fatigue frequently signals an underlying medical or psychological illness.

In most cases, the source of fatigue can be uncovered with a thorough physical exam and a medical history with a particular focus on psychosocial elements combined with a series of blood, urine and saliva tests. More often than not, the women who come into my office complaining that they are "always so tired" have also been told that their fatigue is "all in their mind." Sadly, the tests I run reveal that they have been misdiagnosed and misdirected because they suffering from adrenal exhaustion and an inherent hormonal imbalance. Unfortunately, fatigue has become such a universal symptom that most physicians rarely consider pursuing an adrenal-related diagnosis. The fact that adrenal exhaustion remains commonly undiagnosed is particularly unfortunate because, in most cases, it can be alleviated with a therapeutic regimen that combines lifestyle changes and human-identical hormone replacement.

Why Are We All So Tired?

As you will recall from Chapter 1, the two thumb-sized adrenal glands play a critical role in producing hormones and regulating the sympathetic nervous system. The adrenal glands secrete three hormones in response to stress. They are:

- Epinephrine, the fight-or-flight hormone produced when the body thinks it is being threatened or is in danger.

- Cortisol, the hormone that increases appetite and energy levels while taming the allergic and inflammatory responses of the immune system. Cortisol helps keep the blood sugar at adequate levels to meet the body's demand for energy. When adrenal glands are fatigued, cortisol levels drop lower than normal and the body also suffers from hypoglycemia.

- Dehydroepiandrosterone, or DHEA, which is often referred to as the anti-aging hormone. DHEA has been found to help protect/increase bone density, keep bad cholesterol levels under control, provide a general sense of vitality and energy, aid natural sleep patterns, and improve mental acuity.

Adrenal glands need rest and time to replenish themselves after supporting the body through everyday stresses. Unfortunately, many modern women don't rest or take time to nurture themselves. Instead women today commonly attempt to manage a family, a job, a house, and a budget while striving to stay relatively thin and attractive. Just trying to keep up can be enough to push a woman's adrenal glands into overdrive. When this happens, the hormones that would normally be produced and used sparingly by the body for extreme "fight or flight" situations are drained quickly and unnaturally.

Relentless, debilitating fatigue is a red flag that the adrenal system has been over-stressed and is depleted. The effect of stress is cumulative and can be very toxic. In his groundbreaking book, *Adrenal Fatigue*, Dr. James L. Wilson lists some of the primary factors that can lead to adrenal fatigue. They are as follows:

<u>Lifestyles</u>

- University student
- Mother of two or more children with little or no support from family or friends
- Single parent
- Unhappy marriage
- Extremely unhappy and stressful work conditions
- Self-employed with a new or struggling business
- Drug or alcohol abuser
- Alternating shift work that requires sleep patterns to be frequently adjusted
- All work, little play

<u>Lifestyle Issues</u>

- Lack of sleep
- Poor food choices
- Using food and drinks as stimulants when tired
- Staying up late even when fatigued
- Being constantly in a position of powerlessness

- Constantly driving yourself
- Trying to be perfect
- Staying in no-win situations over time
- Lack of enjoyable and rejuvenating activities

Life Events

- Unrelieved pressure or frequent crises at work and/or home
- Any severe emotional trauma
- Death of a close friend or family member
- Major surgery
- Prolonged or repeated respiratory infection
- Serious burns, including sun burns
- Head trauma
- Loss of a stable job
- Sudden change in financial status
- Relocation without support of friends or family
- Repeated or overwhelming chemical exposure (including drug and alcohol abuse)

Source: *Adrenal Fatigue*, James L. Wilson, N.D., D.C., Ph.D;
Smart Publications, 2001, Petaluma,CA, pg. 17-18.

Based on my experience with and observation of my patients, I would add *divorce* and *caring for an aging parent* to Dr. Wilson's list of life events that can predispose a person to adrenal fatigue.

Over a period of time, if chronic stress is not addressed, the body adapts to adrenal hyper-stimulation and functions in a kind of perpetual fight-or-flight mode. Eventually, the adrenals become exhausted and cortisol levels drop. Fibromyalgia is one example of a condition that can arise when the protective benefits of normal cortisol levels are lost.

The more stress endured, the worse the hormonal problems and the more severe the presenting symptoms. The hallmark symptoms of adrenal dysfunction are stress and fatigue that is not alleviated with sleep; e.g. that "tired all the time" feeling. Other common symptoms include sleep disturbances and/or insomnia, anxiety, depression, increased susceptibility to infections, reduced tolerance for stress, craving for sweet or salt, allergies, chemical sensitivities, and a tendency to feel cold. Studies also validate that a correlation between adrenal dysfunction and symptoms/signs of accelerated aging.

Now, review the above lists one more time. See anyone you know? See yourself? With all the stresses in our lives today, is it really any wonder that our adrenal systems are challenged and we are all so very tired? How can we choose to feel better?

Maybe I Just Need to Take a Nap or a Vitamin

Because feeling tired has become such a common complaint, most people - including physicians - tend to make light of the issue and attempt to bolster lagging energy with a band-aid approach. Time off is a good first step but the adrenal system will not be repaired overnight. Rest is essential for anyone suffering from adrenal fatigue;

however, a single nap or even a short vacation will not allow sufficient time for the adrenal glands to replenish. Conscious choices and lifestyle changes will often be required to eliminate environmental stressors.

A healthy diet will be also key in repairing the adrenal system. Many people who are suffering from adrenal exhaustion have very poor eating habits. They are operating in a fast moving world and, as a result, they too often choose fast food to keep pace. Foods with high fat and high sugar contents provide temporary energy while colas and coffee can provide an immediate perk-up. The problem is that these fast food habits offer very little real nutritional value. When the body is deprived of certain restorative nutrients, the adrenal glands continue to become more fatigued and difficult to stimulate.

Another dietary problem is that people suffering from adrenal exhaustion tend to use snacking in between meals to try and keep their energy from lagging. Not surprisingly, a penchant for snacking usually results in weight gain. According to Dr. Wilson: "the temporary increase in cortisol levels produced by driving the adrenal glands with too much fast food and caffeine causes people with chronically low cortisol to put on weight because even a temporary excess of cortisol causes fat to be deposited around the middle (the spare tire or swallowed-a-beach-ball look)."

Weight gain then tends to cause even more fatigue. The pattern is worsened when women who now feel chunky and sluggish abandon their normal patterns of exercise and physical activity because they are just "too tired to move." This leads to a vicious cycle of unnatural energy stimulation, physical over-performing, adrenal exhaustion, and emotional remorse.

To best support adrenal function, I recommend that my patients choose to avoid foods and beverages that are high in hydrogenated fats, excess caffeine, refined carbohydrates, alcohol, and/or sugar. In addition, I counsel persons suffering from adrenal fatigue that they should not attempt to lose weight via any kind of diet that recommends eschewing one of the major food groups, such as a protein only diet. After reviewing the research related to diet and adrenal fatigue, I recommend eating a balanced diet combining fat, protein, and starchy carbohydrates at every meal to provide a more stable source of energy and put less strain on the body, including the adrenal system. Also, I advise my patients never to skip a meal because low blood sugar further taxes the adrenals.

Vitamin and mineral supplements have value, and I recommend certain ones for my patients suffering from adrenal exhaustion, but they cannot make up for an unhealthy diet or enter the human system and superimpose the normal function of the adrenal hormones.

Breaking the Cycle

In addition to making choices about lifestyle issues and diet, treatment of adrenal exhaustion will usually require some form of human-identical hormone replacement therapy. The stress response, regulated by the adrenal glands, redirects resources and energy away from the reproductive organs. In other words, the ovaries begin to shut down because, when the body is in survival mode, the reproductive system is biologically expendable.

In lay language, adrenal exhaustion not only leads to an imbalance of the stress hormones, e.g. epinephrine, cortisol, and DHEA, but it also catalyzes an imbalance of the sex hormones, e.g. estrogen, progesterone and testosterone. Once an adrenal stress-exhaustion cycle has been established within the body, it will continue until appropriate intervention takes place to restore hormonal balance. Human-identical hormone replacement should be considered a core component of any medical approach to treating adrenal exhaustion.

As in other circumstances where hormonal balance is in question, saliva testing is the first step in establishing a baseline. The body normally secretes the highest amount of cortisol in the morning to get us going, with levels decreasing throughout the day. People with adrenal imbalance will often have abnormally high or low cortisol levels throughout the day. If stress remains high, the adrenals are forced to overproduce cortisol continuously. After a prolonged period of time, the adrenals can no longer keep up with the demand, and total cortisol output plummets, leading to exhaustion.

To obtain an accurate representation of cortisol levels and how the adrenal glands are functioning under stress, it is best to test cortisol levels at least four times throughout a twenty-four hour period. Saliva testing can then chart the extent to which cortisol levels are out of balance. Test results can be used to set a baseline against which the effectiveness of intervention strategies can be measured.

With adrenal fatigue, the body's level of sex hormones - estrogen, progesterone, and testosterone - often fall. Chronic stress can contribute to a deficiency of progesterone. Let's look again at the "Steroid Family Tree" presented in Chapter 1. It is important to understand that, when the body is in the fight-or-flight mode, the biochemical pathway of progesterone can be shifted so that it is used for survival. This means that progesterone can serve as a precursor to the production of more adrenal hormones, rather than

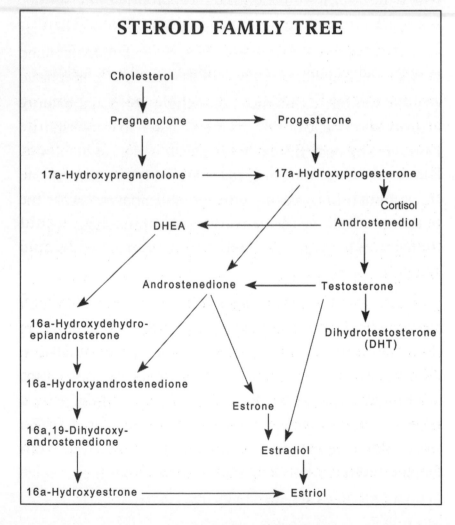

STEROID FAMILY TREE

Cholesterol

Pregnenolone ⟶ Progesterone

17a-Hydroxypregnenolone ⟶ 17a-Hydroxyprogesterone

Cortisol

DHEA ← Androstenediol

Androstenedione ← Testosterone

16a-Hydroxydehydro-epiandrosterone

Dihydrotestosterone (DHT)

16a-Hydroxyandrostenedione

Estrone

16a,19-Dihydroxy-androstenedione

Estradiol

16a-Hydroxyestrone ⟶ Estriol

contributing to all the hormone pathways, in particular balancing and opposing estrogen.

In addition, it is important to note that the adrenal glands also play a role in producing testosterone. Adrenal depletion due to chronic stress may also cause a precipitous drop in testosterone levels. Symptoms of testosterone deficiency may include decreased libido, impaired sexual function, decreased energy overall, decreased sense of well-being, and thinning pubic hair.

Another function of the sex hormones is to act as an antioxidant to help prevent oxidative damage caused by free radicals, those highly unstable molecules that have lost one electron and move through the body scavenging healthy tissues. The lower the sex hormone levels, the more damage there is to tissues, especially under stress. This oxidative damage is one of the key factors in the development of many chronic diseases. Undeterred free radical molecules also catalyze cellular damage that contributes to symptoms and signs associated with rapid aging.

Anti-aging medicine is still in its infancy and much more medical research is needed to validate the anti-aging claims associated with human-growth hormone and DHEA. We do know that the body's production of DHEA declines in tandem with the aging process. For example, at age seventy, most women have only 10% of their peak DHEA levels. Also, supplemental DHEA has been shown to prevent the age-related increase in insulin resistance.

Regardless, human-identical hormone supplementation is an important aspect of any anti-aging strategy. Restoration and maintenance of hormone parameters at youthful levels has been documented to improve health and vitality while also retarding some of the physical and mental signs of aging. Again, saliva testing of hormone levels will be crucial for this approach to be effective.

In most cases of adrenal exhaustion, human-identical hormone replacement will need to encompass both the sex and stress hormones. While human-identical hormone therapy can help address the underlying hormonal issues of deficiency, dominance, and imbalance, it is only part of a treatment plan that embraces the whole woman. Lifestyle choices and dietary changes will also be needed for any woman to heal and break the cycles of physical, mental, and emotional havoc associated with adrenal exhaustion.

Living More and Liking It: Beth's Story (Case Study #4)

The first time I consulted with Beth, (Chapter 2, Case Study #4), I knew that she could be the "poster-child" for adrenal exhaustion. As you may recall, Beth was a thirty-six year old woman who was still regularly menstruating. She had come to see me for her annual exam, but while I was updating her medical history, she had also complained of headaches, extreme fatigue, PMS, and little or no sex drive.

With further questioning, I had learned that Beth was the mother of three-year-old twins and a vice president of a busy public relations firm. As she described her days, I could see why she would feel chronically exhausted. She was always "on" and took very little time to nurture herself or simply to rest. Beth said she drank "a pot of coffee between my shower and my office every morning, then I switch to diet colas and keep one in my hand all day long."

I asked Beth about her diet and she admitted that she dieted continuously to try to manage her weight but still couldn't control frequent binges on sugar and snacks like chips and curly cheese fries. She said that without her snacks, she felt near collapse by mid afternoon.

Because adrenal fatigue is often the cause of premenopause syndrome, I predicted that a saliva test would show that Beth was progesterone deficient. In addition, I knew that we needed to test the levels of Beth's stress hormones, e.g. cortisol and DHEA. I knew that the combination of stress, performance pressures, and poor diet probably had caused Beth's adrenal glands to constantly pump out stress hormones in an effort to keep up with her stressful lifestyle. By now, I was sure that they were more than likely depleted.

Because of the imbalance between Beth's estrogen and progesterone levels, the saliva test confirmed that she was premenopausal. The results of Beth's saliva tests are on the following page. In addition, the findings indicated that her DHEA and cortisol levels were deficient. The fact that her cortisol levels remained low throughout the day validated that Beth was definitely suffering from adrenal exhaustion. Finally, the test results showed that Beth was highly estrogen dominant which was most likely compounding her symptoms of fatigue, headaches, PMS mood swings, and low libido.

Hormone Tested	Within Normal Limits (WNL)	Deficiency (DEF)	Excess (EX)

Estrogen:
  -Estradiol
 	
  -Estriol
 	
  -Estrone
			✔
			
			✔
			
			✔

Progesterone		✔	
Testosterone		✔	
DHEA		✔	
Cortisol		✔	
Progesterone/ Estradiol (Pg/E2) Ratio*		✔	

*The Pg/E2 ratio is a key indicator of hormonal imbalance.

When I shared these findings with Beth, she expressed amazement that there was something actually physically wrong with her. "Gosh, Dr. Randolph," she said, "I had really just begun to accept that being tired all the time was part of aging. Now you tell me that there might be an underlying hormonal imbalance that is causing me to feel this way. I don't like to take a lot of drugs but if you can address my condition in a way that is natural and safe, I am all for it."

Human-identical progesterone cream was the most crucial component in the medical treatment plan I designed for Beth because it would be needed to balance her hormonal profile and oppose the surplus of estrogen now active within her body. I shared with Beth that, if she applied her progesterone cream as directed, her headaches would subside, her energy would increase, her moods and PMS symptoms would improve, and her cravings for caffeine, sweets, and carbohydrates would lessen. Beth looked at me as if I was touting some kind of magical snake oil before she asked dryly, "Dr. Randolph, do you think that your progesterone cream might also do the dishes and fold the laundry?"

I acknowledged to Beth that the potential results of human-identical hormone therapy might seem too good to be true but I asked her to keep an open mind. Sublingual testosterone drops were also recommended. I advised Beth that the potential benefits treating her testosterone deficiency could include a heightened sex drive and higher energy overall.

Then I spoke to Beth about the need to supplement the function of her adrenal glands. "Beth, your saliva tests indicate that you are producing inadequate levels of your adrenal or stress hormones, e.g. cortisol and DHEA. There are several routes for supplementation and I am going to recommend a dosage of each for you to take for the next three months."

I added, "The problem is, Beth, that if you take the supplements for too long, the result can be permanent depression of adrenal function. My goal is to work with you to restore the health and function of your adrenals so that they are eventually able to produce the hormones you need without outside supplements. That will probably require you to make some changes in your lifestyle. Your adrenal glands will not heal with the constant stress that you live with everyday."

With this, Beth sort of rolled her eyes. Given what I knew of her personality, I could guess that she would have preferred a magic pill approach. I wondered how successful this treatment plan would be if she did not address and alter the amount of stress in her life but I knew that, at this point, the next steps were up to her.

Three months later Beth was back in my office. Her saliva test results indicated that the human-identical progesterone cream and testosterone drops had successfully treated the imbalance of her sex hormones: she was no longer estrogen dominant. Her DHEA and cortisol levels were also within normal limits, but then, I knew that Beth was still taking supplements to support her adrenal function. I was interested to learn how Beth's lifestyle changes were, or were not, occurring so that I could appropriately monitor the recovery of her adrenal system.

Beth reported that her headaches were gone completely and that she no longer felt that she was noxiously transformed by PMS once a month. She also told me that her exhaustion was much improved and she had the energy for and the interest in being sexual with her husband. All good news.

"What about your lifestyle, Beth?" I asked. "Any let down from all the stress?"

"Well, Dr. Randolph, there have actually been some radical changes at our house since I saw you last. After you told me about adrenal fatigue, I went home and talked to my husband. I was honestly just going to pretty much blow you off. I mean, no offense, but I really didn't see any way to lighten up. I knew I wouldn't give up my children, my marriage or my home and I honestly really like my job. Besides, I make a lot of money doing what I do."

Beth continued, "My husband, Rick, had other thoughts. He started reading about adrenal exhaustion and became convinced that my constant lack of energy meant that my body's cells were in crisis. He got so worried about what might happen later on, meaning the ongoing deterioration of my health, that he took a stand and told me 'Something's got to give. I have no intention of watching you kill yourself nor do I have any desire to raise these twins on my own'."

"Honestly, I thought he was overreacting but he wouldn't stop harping on things like the fact that I get up at 4:30 every morning, work like I am obsessed and eat junk all day long to keep me going. For a month we did nothing but fight but, then, one day Rick came up with another idea. Though it might sound a bit unconventional to you at your age, Rick has become a house-husband."

I assured Beth that I was not too old to recognize that a man running the home is often a healthy choice for many couples. Beth concurred that this was true for them and went on to explain how it had worked out. "Rick is taking a lesser job with his company so that he can work at home and assume primary responsibility for all that makes our lives go round, like driving the kids to and from school, doing the shopping, maintaining the house, and preparing the meals. Now I can sleep until 7 a.m. and, when I come home in the evening, Rick takes care of dinner so I can spend an hour or so just playing with the twins before I give them a bath. I am beginning to be able to relax and not feel like I am frantically trying to stuff my life into little boxes of time. I even read or write in my journal almost every night before I go to bed and I find that the time calms me so I sleep better."

"Dr. Randolph, I almost feel guilty that I have this choice. I mean, I would have just kept going on until my body wouldn't take me any further. I didn't even know how much I was driving myself into the ground until I slowed down. Thank heaven for Rick." She paused and said, "How do single parents keep up? Or what about women - or men - my age who are taking care of both their children and their parents all at the same time? What about their adrenal systems?"

"Beth," I replied, "I think that adrenal exhaustion is a real epidemic of this millennium; however, you and I can't heal the world - we can only choose to live a lifestyle that will support our health rather than make us sick. I applaud you and Rick for putting your health first, even if it meant making some financial sacrifices. I believe that as more people make healthier choices about how they live and spend their time then perhaps the stressful life with all its bells and whistles will no longer be considered 'hip.' Now, let's talk about how I recommend that we wean you off your adrenal supplements. I think that, over time, your body will be able to do very well on its own."

Chapter 10

Hormone Health during the Reproductive Years

When the medical community and consumers talk about hormone health, the focus is usually on the years right before, during, and after menopause, but the body's production of hormones impacts a woman's health across all her lifecycles. During the reproductive years, most young women are menstruating regularly, and consequently hormonal issues and imbalances can be frequently overlooked until some other kind of physical problem arises. When I was practicing obstetrics and had a practice full of women between twenty and thirty-five, it was an inability to conceive that was most often the first signal. Regular periods are not enough evidence to ensure that the body of a woman in her reproductive years is adequately producing hormones and/or maintaining an optimum hormonal balance.

Hormone Balance and Fertility.... Or Infertility

Both the medical literature and the media highlight infertility as a near epidemic among women in their thirties. There are many causes of infertility. In this chapter, however, we will focus on those causes that are connected to hormone imbalance.

Let's review what should occur naturally to hormone production and balance during a natural menstrual cycle. For a healthy woman in her reproductive years, every 26 to 28 days, the brain signals the ovaries and anywhere from a few to a few hundred eggs begin to mature inside sacs called follicles. After 10 to 12 days, one egg moves to the surface of the ovary, the follicle bursts and the eggs is released into the fallopian tube. From there it journeys into the uterus. The follicle becomes the corpus luteum.

In addition to the eggs produced by the ovaries, the uterus undergoes change during this cycle. The uterine lining becomes thick and engorged with blood. If a fertilized egg becomes implanted in the uterus, this blood will nourish the embryo. If not, the uterine lining will be shed and the monthly menstrual cycle occurs.

Estrogen is the hormone that stimulates the build up of the uterine lining. When the body ovulates, it is estrogen that causes changes in the vaginal mucus to create an environment that is more welcoming for male sperm. Many women track the changes in their vaginal mucus in order to self-monitor their reproductive health.

Watching for the mucus to change to a consistency resembling that of egg whites and monitoring a rise in body temperature is one of the best non-laboratory means of identifying the time of ovulation. Conscious understanding of the body's fertility cycle has been proven to be very effective as a means of contraception, although the diligence and heightened awareness it requires is often daunting to today's busy, modern woman.

Estrogen levels rise during the first ten to twelve days after menstruation and then begin to taper off just as the follicle matures and right before ovulation. Progesterone production dominates the second half of a woman's monthly cycle. Again, progesterone plays a crucial role in preparing the uterus to conceive and sustain the fertilized egg or ovum.

If pregnancy occurs, progesterone levels increase. As the pregnancy progresses, progesterone production shifts from the corpus luteum to the placenta.

The rise and fall of both estrogen and progesterone levels is intimately connected to reproductive health. As a woman ages, her corpus luteum does not manufacture as much progesterone. If the body is estrogen dominant, the ovaries may be producing enough estrogen that the body will appear to have a normal cycle including menstruation, but without sufficient progesterone, the uterine lining will not be adequately prepared for implantation of the ovum.

Hormone imbalance can also negatively impact the composition of the vaginal mucus. Even with normal estrogen levels, if the body is suffering from a deficiency in progesterone, the vaginal environment can be unfriendly towards the sperm, thus preventing fertilization. Progesterone deficiency can also lead to elevated FSH levels, which in turn leads to increased estrogen production. If the follicles are unable to release an egg, no pregnancy is going to occur. Or if the follicle releases the egg, but as it becomes the corpus luteum, it cannot sustain continued progesterone production, the developing embryo will not survive.

Because menstrual cycles can continue without progesterone, most women in their reproductive years aren't aware that it could be the lack of progesterone that is an underlying cause of their inability to conceive. When a young patient fails to conceive, most physicians perform the usual blood tests and check their patient's estradiol and FSH levels. Rarely do most physicians think to check their patient's progesterone levels.

Again, a saliva test can be used to eliminate or illuminate hormone imbalance as a causative factor in infertility. If a deficiency in progesterone is identified, human-identical hormone cream can safely be prescribed. I must underscore that hormone imbalance is just one of the causative factors for infertility.

While I understand the frustration, sadness, and despair common to women who wait every month to discover once again that they are not pregnant, it is very important that women in their reproductive years not attempt to treat an inability to conceive by themselves with over-the-counter progesterone products. Because incorrect timing and use of even human-identical progesterone cream can suppress ovulation, the oversight of a physician who is experienced and knowledgeable in human-identical hormone replacement is a necessity.

Help or Hurt: The Real Story Behind "The Pill"

First, let me say that I still prescribe "the pill" for my patients who have decided that oral contraceptives are their personal choice for birth control. I will add, however, that I am not persuaded that the convenience of using synthetic hormones to suppress ovulation outweighs potential health risks. Let me share with you some facts that I share with my patients so that you too might be better prepared to analyze the data and make your own informed decision regarding the pros and cons of taking birth control pills.

More than 40 years since it was first approved by the U.S. Food and Drug Administration (FDA) in 1960, "the pill" continues to be the most popular and one of the most effective forms of reversible birth control ever invented. According to the Johns Hopkins School of Public Health Population Information Program, more than 100 million women worldwide and 18 million in the U.S. rely on birth control pills today. In the U.S. alone, about 40 different brands are available.

Birth control pills are extremely effective at preventing pregnancy. If used correctly and consistently (that is, no pills are missed and instructions are followed exactly), only 1 in 1,000 women is likely to get pregnant the first year of use. The pill works mainly by preventing ovulation (about 90 to 95 percent of the time). It also works by thickening the mucus surrounding the cervix which helps block the sperm, reduces the risk of pelvic inflammatory disease, and thins the lining of the uterus so that if an egg was fertilized it would have trouble implanting.

Unlike the original oral contraceptives that women took decades ago, there are new low-dose forms of birth control pills that have been shown to have many fewer health risks attached to them. The three most common types of birth control pills are:

- Progestin-only pills: this type of pill contains only synthetic progestin and no estrogen.

- Combined pills: these pills contain a combination of synthetic estrogen and progestin. Combined pills may be monophasic, meaning that each pill in a 21-day pack contains the same amount of synthetic estrogen and progestin, or multiphasic meaning that these pills have different hormone doses throughout the pill-taking schedule.

- Emergency contraceptive pills: these pills are not intended for conventional birth control use but can be helpful preventing pregnancy after unprotected sex. Two products have been approved by the FDA specifically for emergency contraception. One contains both estrogen and progestin (brand name: Preven) and one contains only progestin (brand name: Plan B).

Clinical studies have shown that, in addition to pregnancy prevention, birth control pills can have additional benefits including decreased menstrual blood loss, decreased menstrual cramps and pain, less severe PMS, more regular monthly cycles and decreased acne. Nevertheless, package inserts advise of the following possible side effects: amenorrhea (absence of the monthly period), irregular bleeding, abdominal pain, headaches, nausea and vomiting, breast tenderness, and bloating or weight gain.

According to the National Cancer Institute, the most serious side effect of the pill continues to be an increased risk of cardiovascular disease in certain groups. In addition, women who smoke and/or have certain medical conditions such as a history of blood clots, breast or endometrial cancer should be advised against taking the pill. In 2002, a World Health Organization (WHO) panel examined all recent published data on the risk of stroke and combined oral contraceptive users. The authors concluded that combined oral contraceptive users with a history of migraine may have a two- to four-fold increased risk of stroke over that of nonusers with a history of migraine. Their findings indicated an increased risk of stroke with age.

There is some question as to whether long-term birth control use can later cause infertility or pregnancy problems. The traditional medical response is that they won't. For example, most doctors will tell you that if you take "the pill" from age 20 to 35 and then stop, your chances of getting pregnant will be the same as any other 35 year old. Because of my heightened awareness of the potential dangers associated with synthetic hormones, my personal medical opinion is that we need more research to investigate whether or not chemical birth control puts a woman at greater risk of being infertile in her later years.

Oral contraceptives have also been found to contribute to suboptimal nutrition levels in some women. Women on birth control pills are more likely to be deficient in B vitamin levels, folic acid, and the antioxidant beta-carotene. In addition, oral contraceptives may deplete the body of magnesium and manganese. Women taking "the pill" should supplement their dietary intake with a good multi-vitamin containing B complex and 500 mg of magnesium.

Some of my patients who have gone on "the pill" report to me that they feel moody, depressed and "sort of suspended" within their own body. Oral contraceptives containing synthetic progestin have been shown to interfere to some degree with the brain's production and uptake of serotonin, the chemical within the body which helps regulate mood. The fact that these pills suppress the natural function of a woman's uterus and ovaries may also have emotional and/or psychological impact. Over time, the physical cause and effect of birth control pills may contribute to a woman having feelings of not being connected to the wisdom of her body or to being out of sync with her individual and natural fertility cycles.

Today, I continue to respect my patients' choice when, after reviewing the potential benefits and hazards associated with birth control pills as well as alternative modes for contraception, they still want to walk out of my office with a prescription for "the pill." Still, I remain concerned about the potential long-term health effects of the synthetic hormones in birth control pills. As a result, I continue to research and seek other more natural options. In 2003, I founded the Natural Hormone Institute of America and I have placed the potential use of human-identical hormones for birth control high on our research agenda.

Anorexia and Hormone Imbalance: Toni (Case Study #5)

Let's go back and look again at Toni, the 20 year old patient I introduced to you in Chapter 2 (Case Study #5). Until now, the case studies I have shared with you have illustrated how hormonal imbalance can be treated in ways that lead to happy endings for many patients. This time I have a different story to tell.

As you may recall, Toni had come to see me at the

insistence of her mother who was concerned about Toni's weight loss and absence of periods for more than a year. Toni, however, had told me that she enjoyed being really thin and actually kept up an aggressive exercise schedule that included track and tennis in addition to keeping the pounds off by eating a low fat vegetarian diet.

I confirmed that Toni was suffering from a condition known as amenorrhea, or absence of menstruation. I was also concerned that her body fat was so low. I knew combining the fact that Toni wasn't eating enough calories and nutrients with her propensity for excessive exercise could have deleterious effects. I began to run a battery of tests.

Hormone Tested	Within Normal Limits (WNL)	Deficiency (DEF)	Excess (EX)
Estrogen: -Estradiol		✔	
-Estriol		✔	
-Estrone		✔	
Progesterone		✔	
Testosterone		✔	
DHEA		✔	
Cortisol		✔	
Progesterone/ Estradiol (Pg/E2) Ratio*		✔	

*The Pg/E2 ratio is a key indicator of hormonal imbalance.

As you can see, Toni was deficient in all her sex and stress hormones. Her ovaries were not producing enough estrogen to stimulate her menstrual cycle. Further testing revealed that Toni's FSH levels were too low to foster ovulation. Her adrenal system was essentially depleted. This condition had most likely be exacerbated by her excessive exercise schedule and a diet lacking sufficient nutrients.

Because studies have shown that spinal bone loss occurs in women athletes who have irregular menstrual cycles, I was also concerned that Toni might be at risk for osteoporosis. Despite her young age, a bone density scan indicated that Toni was already suffering from premature bone loss. In fact, Toni's bone density levels were comparable to those of most fifty year old women.

When I shared with Toni her test results and my concerns, she just shrugged. "Dr. Randolph," she replied, "you don't seem to understand that I like my body this way and I intend to stay this thin or thinner. It feels great to me that I can discipline myself and push my body to its limits. You think I need to be menstruating every month but I think menstrual periods are disgusting. And, when you say that I am in the 'reproductive years of my life,' I want to throw up. I never intend to have children so the fact that I am not ovulating is really no problem."

"As far as long term damage to my bones and my organs, I'll try to eat more milk products or take calcium." She continued, "I sort of feel that because you and my mother are from the same generation, you are somehow in cahoots in trying to scare me so that ten years from now I will be some pudgy Junior Leaguer driving three brat children to Chucky Cheese for dinner. That is not who I am or who I want to be. I came in here just to appease my mother but, honestly Dr. Randolph, I have no intention of changing one thing about my life."

I was dismayed with Toni's response, her disdain for her reproductive self as well as her need to put her body under constant surveillance. As I had suspected, Toni's hormone issues were entwined with an eating disorder called anorexia nervosa. I was aware that this condition is present in up to 20 percent of female college students and I knew that, over time, Toni's body-abusing habits could very well have long-term negative health consequences and even put her life at risk.

I gently shared my concerns with Toni. I told her that I would recommend that we work with a nutritionist to help her rehabilitate her metabolism while learning new ways of eating to nurture her body. I also explained that, because her body was lacking in all its essential hormone levels, I wanted to put her on a comprehensive program of human-identical hormone replacement.

Finally, I knew that Toni's case would require a different form of medical expertise than I had to offer. I communicated to Toni in as appropriate manner as possible that I believed that she was suffering from an eating disorder and I would like to refer her to a colleague of mine for psychological counseling. Toni listened to me until I finished speaking and, then without a word, simply stood up and walked out of my office without looking back.

I have not heard from her since.

The tragedy of Toni's case is that it is not that unique. It seems that many women in their reproductive years struggle to accept their bodies and embrace the powerful life-force energy that resides within them. The flow of hormones throughout the body ushers expansion and growth in addition to the possibilities of change, new life stages, as well as species reproduction. For Toni and other women like her, I can only pray that our culture helps to slay those demons driving women to shun the curves of their bodies and/or shut down their "messy" reproductive organs and hormone production.

For any woman, it is expected that the reproductive years will have their travails, but the years of a young woman's life should also be rapt with the wonder of becoming and the celebration of womanhood.

Chapter 11

The Link between Hormones and Breast Cancer

Say the two words "breast cancer" and you will ignite fear in the hearts of most women. These fears are not unwarranted; breast cancer is the most common form of cancer in women and can even be found in men. While heart disease claims more lives than breast cancer, women are generally not as cognizant of their risk for cardiac concerns as they are of their risk for breast cancer. Perhaps the heightened awareness and resulting fear of breast cancer stems from the fact that probably every one of us today knows a woman who has or has had breast cancer. Often that woman was, or is, a mother, sister, close friend, or wife. Breast cancer brings fear to our hearts because, too often, it strikes very close to home.

In 2004, the National Breast Cancer Foundation released the following statistics:

- Every two minutes a woman is diagnosed with breast cancer.

- Every twelve minutes a woman in the United States dies of breast cancer.

- This year more than 200,000 new cases of breast cancer are expected to be diagnosed in the United States.

- When breast cancer is found early, the five-year survival rate is 96%.

- Over 2 million breast cancer survivors are alive in the United States today.

It is not possible to say exactly what causes a woman to develop breast cancer. However, millions of dollars have been spent to research what factors might increase a woman's risk or chance for developing breast cancer in her lifetime. Some well-known risk factors for developing breast cancer include:

- Aging
- Starting menstruation or 'periods' at a relatively early age (before 12 years); and starting menopause or 'the change' at a relatively late age (after 55 years).
- Not having children and/or not breastfeeding.
- Previous diagnosis of breast cancer.
- Drinking alcohol (more than 2 standard drinks a day).
- A family history of breast cancer.

Recent studies released by the American Cancer Society have raised the awareness of two other very potent factors that can increase a woman's risk for developing breast cancer. They are:

- Synthetic hormone replacement therapy (HRT)
- Taking oral synthetic hormone birth control pills (this appears to only increase the risk *during* the period of taking the pill) and
- Obesity

Let's look in depth at how estrogen dominance emerges as a common denominator across most of these risk factors.

The Common Denominators: Hormone Imbalance and Estrogen Dominance

In their book *Are Your Hormones Making You Sick?*, Drs. Eldred and Ava Bell-Taylor clearly describe the role of estrogen and progesterone in normal breast development. In their words: "Estrogen and progesterone are primarily responsible for normal breast development and health. Estrogen has a major influence on breast growth during puberty and also stimulates the growth of the breast ducts while progesterone serves to positively influence the milk producing glands. Another hormone, prolactin, participates in breast development. Pregnancy completes the development of the breast. The influence of increased levels of prolactin, progesterone, and the estrogen (specifically estriol) during pregnancy matures the breast completely."

As we learned in Chapter 5, breast health problems begin when the ratio of one of the sex hormones becomes out of balance with the others. A function of the sex hormone estrogen is to stimulate cell growth and division. In contrast, progesterone functions within the body to stimulate the newly spawned cells to mature and develop. Progesterone also plays a role in promoting normal cell death. Too much estrogen can cause breast cells to multiply faster than normal, and without the balancing effect of progesterone, these cells live longer than they normally would. Uncontrolled growth and extended lifespan of breast cells can lead to breast cancer.

While aging is a known risk factor for breast cancer, it is the hormonal shifts associated with aging that should be identified as the underlying causative agent. Remember, progesterone levels are the first to decline, often beginning as early as a woman's thirties. When progesterone levels decline, the body's balance of estrogen to progesterone is upset. As has been discussed, when the body becomes estrogen dominant, it becomes at risk for many health concerns, including breast and uterine cancers.

When compared to normal breast tissue cells, breast cancer cells show a loss of differentiation and an increased proliferation rate. As cells grow, they are meant to differentiate into the special type of tissue that is encoded in their molecular structure. When breast cells mature at a normal rate, the cells have the time needed to go through their differentiation process. When cells proliferate - or grow - at an abnormally rapid rate, the breast cells have less time to differentiate according to their original genetic coding. These undifferentiated breast cells are permanently damaged with defective growth controls. They are the precursors to cancer. Most breast cancers originate in milk duct epithelial cells.

Women in their mid-thirties to their mid-forties have the highest escalating risk of breast cancer. They are also the age group that is most likely to be highly estrogen dominant. This is very significant. After menopause, when estrogen levels naturally decline, the rate of increase in the risk for breast cancer also drops dramatically. Once again, the data illuminates an interaction between hormone levels - and particularly unopposed estrogen - and breast cancer.

Women who begin to menstruate at an early age are more likely to have hormone levels that begin to shift at an earlier age. In other words, it can be expected that a woman who begins her periods before twelve years of age will be more at risk of becoming estrogen dominant even in her twenties. Similarly, if a woman is late entering menopause, that means that her body is still producing enough estrogen for her to have a monthly period. For both scenarios, estrogen dominance should be investigated as an underlying causative risk factor for breast cancer.

Studies indicate that women who become pregnant before the age of 24 have as much as five times less the risk of breast cancer later in life than women who wait until they are 30 years or older to have their first child. Hormone shifts that occur in pregnancy result in the complete development of a woman's breast. In addition, the hormones of pregnancy and lactation develop and differentiate the breast tissue in ways that are highly protective. It is important to recognize that progesterone is the dominant hormone during pregnancy and that progesterone is the hormone that encourages cells to differentiate and to die when they are supposed to.

The reason why women who do not have children and/or do not breastfeed are at higher risk for developing breast cancer is most likely due to the fact that their breast tissue has never gone through the cell differentiation that occurs with pregnancy and lactation. As a result, the breast tissue of these women has not been afforded the extra protection from the natural flux of hormones associated with gestation and lactation. For women who have had children and/or breastfed, the hormone balancing action of an increase in progesterone during pregnancy provides them with extra protection against breast cancer.

Women with a previous diagnosis of breast cancer have been found to have a five times greater risk for developing breast cancer again in the same or opposite breast. If the body is chronically estrogen dominant, removal of the cancerous breast cells only removes the result but does not address the underlying causative agent. Think about it. It stands to reason that if the body's estrogen levels remain dominant and unopposed, they will continue to foster the rapid cell proliferation and growth that spawned the first cancer. As will later be discussed in greater detail, hormone balancing should be integral to the treatment and recovery plan for breast cancer survivors.

Estrogen dominance is also tied to alcohol consumption. One of the functions of the liver is to process estrogen out of the body. When the liver is stressed by alcohol, it becomes inefficient in metabolizing and eliminating estrogen so the body has chronically higher levels of estrogen than it would otherwise. Therefore, women who consume more than two alcoholic drinks a day are at greater risk of being estrogen dominant and women who are estrogen dominant are at a higher risk for developing breast cancer.

Now, look again at the list of risk factors. Hormone imbalance and particularly estrogen dominance are linked to five out of six well-known risk factors. The premise here is that too much estrogen can cause cancer, while progesterone, as a hormone-balancing agent, can help prevent breast cancer. If this is fundamentally true, and I am convinced that it is, it is frightening to consider how often it is overlooked in the conventional approach to breast health and breast cancer treatment.

What about Genetics?

Genetics can play a role in the development of breast cancer; however, while a history of breast cancer in the family may lead to an increased risk, most breast cancers are diagnosed in women with no family history. A relatively small percentage of breast cancers, 5 to 7 percent, is attributable to inherited mutations of the BRCA1 gene. These are typically familial, early onset cancers. BRCA1 is a tumor suppressor gene located on the long arm of the chromosome 17. Tumor suppressor genes play a role in regulating cell growth. When one copy of the BRCA1 is inherited in a defective form, a woman is predisposed for breast cell proliferation. Women who carry a mutation in the BRCA1 gene have an 80% risk of breast cancer and a 40% risk of ovarian cancer by the age of seventy.

Before testing for the BRCA1 gene can occur, a thorough family history should be taken. Currently, testing is only recommended for women with two or more first-degree relatives (mother, sister, daughter) who have suffered from breast and/or ovarian cancer. These relatives should actually be tested first. If they have the mutation, then others within the gene pool might be at risk. If they do not have the mutation, then genetics can be eliminated as a predisposing factor for breast cancer.

It is important to note that positive or negative test results do not provide black and white answers. While a positive test result indicates an increased risk for developing breast cancer, it does not mean that breast cancer will be inevitable. Likewise, a negative test result does not mean that a woman can't get breast cancer. She is just as much at risk from other factors as any other woman; she just won't develop breast cancer as a result of a genetic predisposition.

When a mutant gene does exist, estrogen dominance is not the driving force behind the risk for developing breast cancer. There is, however, an interesting analogy between the function of the BCRA1 gene and progesterone. When the BCRA1 gene is present in its non-mutant form it serves to help regulate cell growth. When progesterone is in balance with estrogen, it also functions to help regulate cell growth. While their functions are not metabolically linked, it is interesting to note the similar cancer-protecting effects of both the BRCA1 gene and the sex hormone, progesterone.

Synthetic HRT and Estrogen Dominance: A Very Toxic Duo

As I stated in the Introduction, it was after observing a higher incidence of fibrocystic breasts and breast tumors in my patients on synthetic HRT that I began to research and investigate clinical alternatives for treating my patients suffering from symptoms associated with menopause or hormonal imbalance. Today, I am even more stalwart in my medical opinion regarding the dangers of synthetic HRT. The good news is that the medical evidence is mounting to substantiate my position. The bad news is that too many women have been, and unfortunately still are, prescribed synthetic HRT. By "following doctor's orders," these women often unknowingly increasing their risk for developing breast cancer.

For many years, the medical community at large has chosen to ignore the evidence that synthetic HRT increases a woman's risk for developing breast cancer. As a result of the release of the WHI study's findings, it is now more difficult for physicians to ignore or undermine the studies linking synthetic HRT to risk of breast cancer, later diagnosis, and more abnormal mammograms.

According to an article in the June 25, 2003, issue of *The Journal of the American Medical Association* (JAMA), even relatively short-term use of combined estrogen plus progestin has been proven to be associated with a higher incidence of breast cancer. The researchers wrote: "The breast cancers diagnosed in women in the HRT group were more likely to be in an advanced stage than the placebo group. These results suggest that invasive breast cancers developing in women receiving synthetic estrogen plus progestin may have an unfavorable prognosis."

As discussed in earlier chapters, there are two primary reasons why synthetic HRT can have such a toxic, and potentially carcinogenic, effect on the body. First, synthetic hormones are molecularly different than the hormones they were designed to replace. The synthetic hormone "key" doesn't exactly fit the human body's hormone receptor "lock." Clinical studies have proven that even a slight difference in molecular structure can initiate a biochemical response at the cellular level that, ultimately, will result in serious and deleterious effects within the body.

The relationship between estrogen dominance and synthetic HRT is the second red flag. The traditional medical community has been trained to treat symptoms associated with menopause and hormone imbalance with *more estrogen.* This is erroneous thinking. As you know from what you have read thus far in this book, most of the symptoms associated with menopause and hormone imbalance result from a progesterone deficiency resulting in a condition of estrogen dominance.

Treating estrogen dominance with more estrogen in effect just adds more negative fuel to the fire. Without progesterone, estrogen is unbounded in its ability to promote a cancerous condition by stimulating breast cell growth. It is important to recognize that the negative consequences associated with too much estrogen occur regardless of whether the estrogen added into the body is synthetic or human-identical.

The pharmaceutical industry has attempted to offset the cancer-promoting role of estrogen by using synthetic progestin in many formulations of synthetic HRT. While the rationale of balancing unopposed estrogen has merit, the use of a synthetic version of progesterone does not. Let me be clear: progestin's molecular structure is not identical to progesterone. In the body, it is another key that doesn't exactly fit its hormone receptor lock. Some of the synthetic progestins can have estrogenic activity causing persistent stimulation of breast tissues. *The consequences can be deadly.*

Oral contraceptives, or birth control pills, are another form of synthetic HRT. The 'pill' is chemically designed to suppress ovulation. As a result, the body's natural hormone rhythms are masked. In addition, the synthetic estrogens and progestins in oral contraceptives have the potential to assault immature breast cancer cells so that they become more vulnerable to cancer-causing agents.

As Dr. Lee pointed out in his book *What Your Doctor May Not Tell You About Breast Cancer*, birth control pills are also known to deplete a number of vitamins, including vitamin B6 and folic acid. Folic acid is essential for protecting the DNA from damage, which is more likely when excessive amounts of hormones are present. A deficiency in these vitamins is also known to contribute to cervical dysplasia, and it's reasonable to expect that their deficiency may also contribute to excessive proliferation of breast cancer cells.

Many women are unprepared to use a birth control method other than birth control pills. For my patients who choose to remain on oral contraceptives, I see it as my role as their physician to be on the alert for the possibility that 'the pill' has the potential to increase the breast cells' proliferation and vulnerability to carcinogens. In these cases, after advising my patient of my concerns, I ask them to be highly vigilant regarding other side effects such as headaches, blood clotting, or exacerbated PMS. My theory is that these less life-threatening symptoms can be the first signal that the body's hormone receptors are rejecting the molecular structure of the synthetic estrogen and progestins.

Fat → Hormone Imbalance → Breast Cancer

According to research released in early 2004 by the American Cancer Society, the amount of weight a woman gains after 18 is a strong signal as to whether she will get breast cancer later in life. Researchers found that women who gained twenty to thirty pounds after high school graduation were 40 percent more likely to get breast cancer than women who kept the weight off. Women who gained seventy or more pounds doubled their risk of developing breast cancer.

As we established in earlier chapters, fat tissues make estrogen, specifically estrone. Estrone negatively fosters breast cell proliferation more than the other two estrogens, estradiol and estriol. In addition, when fat is metabolized, free radicals are produced. The more free radicals, the greater damage to tissue at the cellular level and, consequently, the higher incidence of cancer.

One of the problems that I regularly see is that, when a woman's hormones are out of balance, her metabolism and thyroid function are upset. This makes it more difficult for her to lose weight even when sticking to a nutritional regimen that should be conducive to weight loss. In these cases, I find that a human-identical hormone replacement regimen is required to reestablish the body's natural equilibrium. Most often, human-identical progesterone replacement is the most seminal component the hormone regimen.

In concert with hormone imbalances, dietary and lifestyle issues must be addressed in order for the weight to stay off. When a woman consumes more calories than she needs to fuel her energy needs, those calories are stored as fat. Again, the fat increases estrogen levels. When energy needs exceed caloric intake, both total body fat and estrogen levels decline.

Our fast-paced culture lends itself to the consumption of empty calories. Women are constantly on the run, and to sustain themselves, they often reach for colas, pretzels, cookies, bagels and/or a candy bar. These refined carbohydrates have little nutritive value. In fact, they are detrimental to the balance of fatty acids in the body and are linked to insulin resistance and the disruption of normal hormone production in the brain and ovaries. Over time, the diet itself can foster an overproduction of estrogen and an underproduction of progesterone.

I recommend that my patients who are overweight commit to eating a balanced diet while also limiting their caloric intake. I suggest that my patients avoid consuming excess animal fats while I emphasize the curative value of increasing their intake of vegetables and fruits that have been shown to be protective against cancer. Many studies have shown that plant chemicals, or phytochemicals, have an effect at the cellular level that serves to inhibit cancer initiation, promotion and progression.

What we eat truly can reduce breast cancer risk. For instance, cruciferous vegetables such as broccoli and cauliflower have been shown to remove carcinogens from cells by boosting enzyme activity. Remember from Chapter 5 that estrogens can go down one of two pathways: the 16-hydroxy pathway or the 2-hydroxy pathway. The 16-

hydroxy pathway is the beginning of the cascade that ends up forming DNA-damaging catechol and quinone estrogens while the 2-hydroxy is the safer pathway. Phytochemicals from the cruciferous vegetables encourage estrogens down the 2-hydroxy pathway. Just as exciting is the fact that the phytochemicals in these same vegetables have the power to help a precursor to estrogen break up into a benign, rather than cancer-causing, form.

There is more good news. Citrus fruits contain flavonoids that can prevent cancer-causing hormones from latching onto a cell. Hot peppers contain capsaicin that has the capacity to keep toxic molecules from attaching to the DNA. Soybeans contain genistein that functions within the body to inhibit growth of blood vessels to cancer cells, thereby retarding or eliminating breast tumor growth.

Finally, I recommend that my patients who are overweight and estrogen dominant take Calcium D-glucarate. This particular vitamin supplement helps the body excrete excess estrogen through the bowel. Calcium D-glucarate is so potent that when it was given to rats specially bred to have a 100 percent risk of cancer, only 56 percent got it. And the animals that did get cancer had 87.5 percent fewer tumors than normal. In fact, Calcium D-glucarate is so promising as an adjunct therapy that the NIH is studying its use in women at risk for developing breast cancer.

Xenohormones Contribute to Breast Cancer Risk

Scientists have estimated that 50 to 95 percent of

cancers are caused by diet and environment. As you may recall from discussions in earlier chapters, xenohormones are petrochemicals found in our everyday environment that can disrupt health hormone production and function. These petrochemicals can include pesticides, herbicides, paint, solvents, glues, and even noxious fumes from fabrics and carpets. Some of the highest levels come from detergents that are used in commercial enterprises and end up in municipal water supplies. Many of the xenohormones mimic the action of estrogen once they get into the body, including triggering cancer. DDT is one of these chemicals commonly recognized for its carcinogenic effect; atrazine, the common herbicide used on corn, is another.

Xenohormones also migrate into foods from packaging. Specifically, plastics have the potential to increase breast cancer risk. The plastic wrap around purchased vegetables, fruits, and meats contains those dangerous estrogen mimics. So does the plastic bottle holding that pure water you are drinking to promote your health. The xenohormones leach from the plastic into the foods and drinks we consume everyday and are most likely contributing to the epidemic rise in breast cancer.

The Journal of Applied Toxocology recently released a study linking deodorants and antiperspirants to breast cancer risk. Previous studies, including a study of more than 1,500 women that was published in the *Journal of the National Cancer Institute*, have disputed that topically applied underarm cosmetics could have a cancer causative effect. While the controversy continues to rage, it has been proven that chemicals can be absorbed through the skin and, if they accumulate in sufficient quantities, they act weakly like estrogen. The degree of risk has yet to be determined.

If you think about it, it is mind-boggling how many of the estrogen mimics the average person is exposed to every day. Although xenohormones do not resemble the estrogen molecule in chemical structure, they nevertheless cause potent estrogenic activity once in the body. First, they can bond with estrogen receptors like a woman's estrogen-estradiol. After attaching to a hormone receptor, they then transmit a message that tells the breast cells to proliferate at an unnatural rate. Secondly, some xenohormones have been shown to release a chemical that actually promotes tumor growth. As they stimulate breast cancer cell growth, xenohormones contribute to several mechanisms that support and sustain the cancer.

Chemicals are part of our lives, but I suggest that we all do what we can to avoid xenohormones. Here is a list of opportunities that I frequently share with my patients:

- Don't purchase foods wrapped in plastic.
- When at all possible, choose organic products and free-range meats.
- Throw away all pesticides, herbicides, and fungicides, and replace them with organic or natural equivalents.
- Abstain from using cosmetics that have solvents in them, such as fingernail polish remover, and consider an alternative to hairspray, such as an organic hair mousse.

- Avoid microwaving food in plastic containers or covered in plastic wrap.
- Drink filtered water out of a glass container, not a plastic bottle.

Applying all these choices may or not be realistic given a person's lifestyle. However, women who are committed to doing everything they can to reduce their risk of breast cancer are typically grateful to have information that can help them become more conscious of how their choices may or may not unknowingly put them at greater risk. I believe that any steps a woman takes to intentionally protect breast health will, over time, prove to be beneficial.

Progesterone Promotes Breast Health

Naturally-occurring progesterone and human-identical progesterone can serve to neutralize the cancer-promoting properties of estrogen while also instigating many other beneficial effects within the body. Unfortunately, while the medical community widely acknowledges that too much estrogen in the body can serve as a catalyst for the development of breast cancer, there is still some skepticism regarding the cancer-protective attributes of progesterone. As a physician and pharmacist, it amazes me that the pharmaceutical industry has successfully promoted the use of progestin, e.g. a synthetic form of progesterone, to offset the cancer-promoting role that estrogen plays within the body.

Why should any physician be duped into believing that a synthetic product does not come with its own health issues and side effects? Why not prescribe and replace a hormone with one that has the exact same molecular structure as the one originally produced by the ovaries? Why not trust that Mother Nature knew what she was up to when she set the blueprint for our hormones within our DNA?

As Dr. Schwartz so succinctly said in her book *The Hormone Solution*, breast cancer is a hormone dependent cancer. Continuous exposure to high levels of unopposed estrogen can increase a woman's chances of getting breast cancer. Women can be exposed to too much estrogen when:

- It is out of balance with progesterone.
- They receive it in the form of synthetic estrogen replacement therapy; HRT.
- Or when they are exposed to toxic xenoestrogens in our environment.

Source. Ericka Schwartz, M.D., *The Hormone Solution*, 2002, pg 146

As a conventionally trained physician, I, too, was initially very skeptical that my medical school training had failed to teach me about the health benefits of progesterone. It seemed absurd to me that many of the brightest clinical and research minds in the country had somehow overlooked something so seemingly obvious and simple as hormone balancing. As I said in the Introduction, I began my own search for alternatives because of my concern about the higher incidence of breast cancer and fibrocystic breasts that I observed in my patients on synthetic HRT. It was through contact with Dr. John Lee that I was given the scientific data I needed to recognize the health benefits of progesterone as a hormone-balancing agent. As I have said, my exposure to and mentoring from Dr. Lee changed my life and my practice forever.

Today, I applaud my physician peers who are open-minded enough to consider that progesterone can have cancer-protective benefits but who are analytical enough to be true stewards of their patients' care and treatment. I really appreciate it when a physician says to me: "Sounds good, but I won't expose my patients to anything that has not been clinically proven to be both safe and effective. Show me the data."

Here is the bad news: most of the studies on hormone replacement – including WHI and others recently cited in the media – have been conducted using synthetic hormones. The medical community is right to demand more long-term epidemiological studies of the health effects, benefits and/or concerns associated with human-identical hormone therapies. This need was the primary motivator for my foundation of The Natural Hormone Institute of America in 2003. One of the critical goals of The Institute will be to foster and support research evaluating human-identical hormone therapies.

In the meantime, there is still good news. While not as voluminous as the studies investigating synthetic HRT, there are still many studies offering solid clinical evidence as to the cancer-protecting properties of progesterone. For starters, please read carefully the studies cited in the following excerpt from Dr. Lee's book *What Your Doctor May Not Tell You About Breast Cancer*.

The Relationship of Sex Hormones to Breast Cancer

Most experienced clinicians understand very well that estrogen is a promoter of breast cancer, and they also understand that progesterone balances or opposes undesirable side effects of estrogen. For reasons that aren't entirely clear, conventional medicine has ignored the cancer-protective effects of progesterone in treating breast cancer despite many studies that offer solid evidence.

Even though progestins (synthetic progesterone) are used in hormone replacement therapy to offset or oppose the cancer-promoting role of estrogen in endometrial cancer, progesterone has not been widely recognized for its similar role in breast cancer. And yet there are studies that clearly establish this relationship. As long ago as 1966 H. P. Leis reported treating 158 menopausal women (11 percent with a strong family history of breast cancer) with both estrogen and progesterone therapy for up to 14 years; none of the patients developed breast cancer.

In rodent studies by A. Inoh, the protective effect of progesterone or tamoxifen was investigated in estrogen-induced mammary cancer. The ovaries of the rats were removed. Rats given estradiol had a high rate of mammary cancer. However, if tamoxifen or progesterone was given simultaneously with estradiol, fewer tumors appeared, and the ones that did were smaller and less likely to spread. Tamoxifen, a patent drug, has been introduced as a standard breast cancer treatment in conventional medicine, but progesterone has been ignored. Given the toxicity of Tamoxifen, we believe it is a tragedy that progesterone has been ignored in this context.

The action of estradiol and progesterone on cell multiplication (proliferation) in breast cells was beautifully demonstrated in an important 1995 study by K. J. Chang and coworkers. It tested the effects of transdermal (via the skin) hormone applications on normal human breast duct cells, from which cancer is known to rise, in health young women planning to undergo minor breast surgery for benign breast disease.

In this study the women were divided into four groups and began using one of the creams on their breasts 10 to 13 days before breast surgery:

- Group A applied estradiol cream (1.5 mg) daily.

- Group B applied progesterone cream (25 mg) daily.

- Group C applied a combination of estradiol and progesterone (half doses each) daily.

- Group D applied a placebo cream.

At surgery, biopsies were obtained for measuring estradiol and progesterone concentractions, and for tests of cell proliferation rates. In addition, blood plasma hormone levels were measured. Following surgery the breast tissue, about the size of a marble, was divided in half. One part was sent to a pathology laboratory for viewing under a microscope to determine how the hormones affected the growth rate of the breast cells; the remainder was sent to an endocrinology laboratory to determine how much hormone was taken up by the tissue.

Results from the endocrinology laboratory revealed that in those women treated with just estradiol, the concentration of estradiol in the breast tissue was 200 times greater than those not treated with it (placebo gel). Breast tissue concentrations of progesterone were 100 times greater in women who had used progesterone than the placebo. These findings clearly demontrate that both hormones are well absorbed transdermally (through the skin) and accumulate in target tissues in the same manner as endogenous (made in the body) hormones. This is important because it's common for conventional doctors to claim that transdermal progesterone isn't absorbed.

The effect of these hormones on cell proliferation rates was equally clear. Estradiol increased the cell proliferation rate by 230 percent, whereas progesterone *decreased* it by more than 400 percent. The estradiol-progesterone combination cream maintained the normal proliferaton rate. Again, this is clear evidence that unopposed estradiol stimulates hyperproliferation of breast cells and progesterone protects against this.

When progesterone is used transdermally, blood tests don't show a measurable rise, and this is why so many doctors believe it isn't absorbed. What's important to take away from this study is the fact that progesterone levels rose dramatically in the breast cells of women using transdermal progesterone, and this proves that progesterone is well absorbed when applied to the skin. The blood tests show no measurable increase of progesterone concentration, however. This is an excellent illustration of the fact that blood testing can't be reliably used to determine the bioavailability level of progesterone when it's delivered through the skin, because very little bioavailable progesterone is carried in the blood plasma, which is what's measured in a standard blood test.

Dr. Zava has noted both in carefully controlled clinical studies and in daily testing of thousands of saliva samples that this same dosing of progesterone (about 20 to 30 mg) results in a remarkable increase in salivary progesterone, as much as 10 to 50 times, more closely reflecting what K. J. Chang and colleagues found in breast tissue uptake of these hormones. Two studies recently reported from Australia confirm that topical progesterone results in very little increase in serum progesterone but a remarkable increase in saliva levels of progesterone.

Excerpted from *What Your Doctor May Not Tell You About Breast Cancer*, (2002). John R. Lee, M.D., David Zava, Ph.D., Virginia Hopkins, M.A. pg 101-105.

Help and Hope

There is good reason to consider that balancing estrogen with progesterone or human-identical progesterone has the potential to decrease a woman's risk for breast cancer. Both women consumers and physicians treating women bear responsibility for educating themselves on the science of how progesterone works within the body to have a cancer-protecting effect. As to what choices are made to promote and preserve breast health, that responsibility will ultimately lie with each individual woman.

For women who have previously lived in fear of breast cancer and have felt that it was just a matter of time until they, too, were diagnosed, there is help. For women who have already suffered an assault on their lives as a result of this ravaging disease and believe that any day now "the other shoe will fall," there is hope. If the medical community can actively begin to examine the cancer-preventing benefits of hormone balancing and particularly human-identical progesterone replacement, I firmly believe that I will live to see the day when breast cancer will no longer be diagnosed in epidemic proportions in the United States. As a physician, a son, a brother, and a father, I look forward to that future.

Chapter 12

Men Have Hormones Too: Understanding Andropause

I frequently have female patients who, after having been successfully treated with human-identical hormones, ask me if it is possible that the men in their lives might also be susceptible to hormone imbalance. The answer is a definitive "Yes!"

Menopause Is Not Just for Women

While most men continue to think that menopause is a "woman's thing," the fact is that - as men age - they too experience a decline in the hormones that promote masculinization. By the time men are between the ages of 40 and 55, they will begin to experience a phenomenon similar to women's menopause, called andropause. Unlike women, men do not have a clear-cut signpost such as the cessation of menstruation to mark this transition. Both, however, are distinguished by a drop in hormone levels: progesterone and estrogen in women and testosterone in men. Physical, mental and emotional changes associated with andropause tend to emerge very gradually. Symptoms may include lethargy, urinary problems, erectile dysfunction, decreased physical agility, and depression.

Andropause is not a new condition. It was first described in the medical literature in the 1940's but, until recently, it was not a topic of conversation for either male patients or their physicians. The unpleasant side effects associated with hormone imbalance were simply written off as an unavoidable consequence of aging. Two factors have helped to increase awareness that men, too, may suffer from symptoms related to hormone imbalance.

Demographics are the first contributing factor. There is literally an explosion occurring right now in the number or men over the age of 45. These baby-boomer males have the mindset of living a long, productive, and enjoyable life. They have no patience when, during what they regard as the prime of their lives, they begin to experience a loss of energy, mental acuity, physical strength, and/or sexual stamina. Suddenly, these male consumers are asking questions and demanding that the medical community come up with some answers.

The advent of Viagra, the top-selling prescription drug with gross sales of $521 million in 2003, made male sexual health a topic of national conversation. Now that television features well-known men like Bob Dole openly talking about Viagra and Mike Ditka endorsing Levitra, men who found it difficult to even admit that they had a problem with erectile dysfunction are comparing notes and results with their buddies on the golf course.

The women in their lives are also speaking up. Every week in my practice at least a half dozen of my female patients initiate a conversation with me about their husband's or lover's change in libido, sexual performance, overall energy, and moods. It is no longer taboo to discuss the physical and emotional changes men go through as they enter the second phase of their lives.

I find that my female patients are grateful to learn that they aren't the only ones going through "the change." Moreover, they are relieved to learn that there is most likely a medical reason for why the men in their lives might be more irritable, tired all the time, and lacking the enthusiasm for the things that previously gave them joy and stirred them up. Finally, both these women and their partners are elated to learn that treatment with human-identical testosterone can help restore quality of life.

What Does Testosterone Have to Do with Andropause?

Testosterone is the principal male hormone. It is the primary androgenic hormone and is responsible for normal growth and development of male sex organs and maintenance of secondary sex characteristics. Testosterone is the hormone that stimulates the development of the male secondary characteristics after puberty, causing growth of the beard and pubic hair, development of the penis, and voice changes. Testosterone also aids in growth, muscular development, masculine body contour of the adult male, libido and maturation of the sperm. Finally, testosterone functions to accelerate muscle build up, increase the formation of red blood cells, speeds up regeneration, and helps to reduce the recovery time needed after injuries.

Testosterone is produced by the Leydig cells in the male testes. Using cholesterol as a base, the testes produce between 4 and 10 mg of testosterone per day. During puberty, testosterone levels are at their lifetime peak. They begin to decline around the age of 25.

For younger men, infertility is often a first sign of post-pubertal testosterone deficiency. The sperm will not mature because the body is not producing enough testosterone. As a man ages, however, the clinical symptoms and signs may evolve slowly and subtly, making them more difficult to detect. Too often, men in their 40's or 50's will simply assume that they are "no longer a spring chicken" and just write off the physical, emotional, and mental symptoms of testosterone deficiency. This is not only a sad consequence for a man's quality of life but, if a testosterone deficiency remains undiagnosed and untreated, it can have other longer-term and more severe health effects.

Andropause and Osteoporosis

In a healthy individual, bone tissue is constantly being broken down and rebuilt. In an individual with osteoporosis, more bone tissue is lost than is regenerated. We've addressed how women frequently suffer from osteoporosis after menopause if the balance of estrogen, progesterone and testosterone is not reestablished. In men, testosterone is thought to be the most essential pivot in maintaining the body's balance for bone density.

Unfortunately, with advancing age and declining testosterone levels, men, like women, seem to demonstrate a similar pattern of risk for developing osteoporosis. Between the ages of 40 and 70 years, male bone density typically falls by 15 percent. Studies estimate that approximately one in eight men over the age of 50 actually has some degree of osteoporosis. Low bone density puts one at risk for frequent fractures, associated pain, and in more severe cases, loss of mobility and independence. Wrists, hips, spines, and ribs are the most commonly affected.

Andropause and Cardiovascular Risk

There are a few clinical trials that seem to suggest that a man's risk of atherosclerosis (hardening of the arteries) increases as his testosterone levels diminish with age. While the research is not complete, the clinical findings point to a possible association between low testosterone levels and an increase in cardiovascular risk for men. Additional clinical trials will be required before the medical community can scientifically identify a cause and effect relationship between testosterone levels and heart health.

The Benefits of Human-Identical Testosterone Replacement

In many instances, human-identical testosterone replacement in men with andropause can be highly effective and beneficial. It's not for every man, of course, even those who show symptoms may have other health problems at the root of their health concerns. Before I will treat a male patient with testosterone therapy I require a medical and medication history, a physical exam, and a directed laboratory evaluation. Testosterone therapy is most definitely contraindicated in men who have or have had prostrate or breast cancer.

To establish a baseline, I order a serum blood or saliva test to measure free serum testosterone, as well as levels of progesterone and estradiol. Testing is best done in the morning. I also do a bone density screen on these male patients to identify any evidence of bone density loss. In addition, I perform a digital rectal exam to check for an enlarged prostate or the presence of a mass. Finally, I order a prostatic specific antigen (PSA) titer, a tumor marker for prostrate cancer. A PSA level greater than 3.5 is an indicator of prostrate cancer.

When human-identical hormone replacement therapy is indicated, a safe general principle is to mimic the body's normal concentrations, e.g. add back in what is missing or has been lost. The ultimate goal is to normalize the male physiology. Ideal testosterone replacement therapy produces and maintains physiologic serum or saliva concentrations of the hormone and its active metabolites without significant side effects or safety concerns.

Several different types of testosterone replacement are currently marketed, including tablets, injectables and transdermal creams. I typically prescribe 1% testosterone either in a topical gel form or sublingual drops, depending on my patient's preference.

Almost all of the male patients for whom I have prescribed human-identical testosterone replacement have had a positive response. The reported positive outcomes include:

- Improvement in mood and sense of well-being
- Increased mental and physical energy
- Decreased anger, irritability, sadness, tiredness

- Decreased nervousness / Increased calm
- Improved quality of sleep
- Improved libido and sexual performance
- An increase in lean body mass and a decline in fat mass
- An increase in muscle strength
- Stabilized or increased bone density

These effects are often noted within three to six weeks.

For men who desire fertility at some time in their life, hormonal therapy directed at enhancing spermatogenesis (production of the sperm) may offer them that opportunity. After fertility therapy is deemed a success or failure, it is recommended that the patient resume a hormone replacement regimen designed to maintain an equilibrium of testosterone levels.

What Happened to Jake?

Jake came to see me at the insistence of his wife, Pat, who had been my patient for more than twenty years. I had delivered both of their children, a boy and a girl, so I had had the opportunity to meet Jake in that context, but today was different. Jake came in through the back door so as not to be seen by all the women sitting in my waiting room. I understood his reticence so I had instructed my staff to accommodate his need for added privacy. Now, sitting face-to-face, Jake looked as if he wished he could crawl into a hole in the floor.

"Well, Dr. Randolph," he started, "I guess Pat told you that I just don't want to 'do it' anymore. You know, I am not even sure why. I love Pat; my goodness, she has been my best friend for over thirty years. And, I tell you, she still looks great with all that working out she does and playing tennis. It's just that at 54 years old, I would rather just sit on the couch in the evening and then just go asleep. Maybe I am just getting old and everything in my life will be downhill from here on."

Jake continued, "I told Pat that I wouldn't blame her if she'd rather just put me out to pasture, but instead, she asked me if I would come see you. Well, I have to tell you, that sort of blew me away. I mean me coming to see my wife's gynecologist sounds like I am really a desperate case but I guess the good news is that she didn't ask me to go see one of those candy-ass therapists that some of my buddies' wives have made them go to."

"Jake," I responded, "I certainly understand why you might be uncomfortable coming to see a gynecologist but, if it helps, I have several male patients that I treat and see regularly. Still, if you would prefer, I can refer you to another physician - perhaps an internist, endocronoligist or urologist - to discuss your concerns with. Pat thought it might be beneficial for you to see me after she read an article on male hormone replacement. As I am sure you are aware, Pat has personally had a very positive response to the regimen of human-identical hormone therapies that I prescribed for her almost a year ago. Since you are already here, let's see if I can at least make your trip to my office worth your time and trouble. If it is alright with you, I would like to chat with you for a few minutes and ask you three or four questions."

"Sure, what the heck," Jake responded. "Now that I am here, I might as well get my money's worth. What do you want to know?"

In working with men who I suspect are suffering from a possible hormonal deficiency or imbalance, I use a derivation of the following questionnaire developed by John Morley, M.D.:

1. Do you have a decrease in libido (sex drive)?

2. Do you have lack of energy?

3. Do you have a decrease in strength and/or endurance?

4. Have you lost height?

5. Have you noticed a decreased "enjoyment of life"?

6. Are you sad and/or guilty?

7. Are your erections less strong?

8. Have you noticed a recent deterioration in your ability to play sports?

9. Are you falling asleep after dinner?

10. Has there been a recent deterioration in your work performance?

Answering yes to questions 1 or 7, or to any other three questions consititutes a positive result.

With Jake, I thought it might be less threatening if I started by asking him to tell me about his work. "You know, Dr. Randolph," he responded, "I am Senior Vice President of New Product Development for a large HMO based here in Florida. I have always been regarded as the 'rising star' in the executive team and my work has even been recognized nationally. Recently, however, I feel strained to just sit through meetings. I don't have any pep or enthusiasm for the projects I am in charge of. It's as if I can't come up with any new ideas or strategies."

"What is worse," Jake went on, "is that, when I delegate a problem or need to my staff, I am actually resentful when they come up with great solutions or cutting-edge ideas. I get pretty unreasonable. My administrative assistant, Donna, who has worked for me for the past seventeen years told me I was no fun to work for any more. She also told me, that in the last year or so, I was becoming unreasonable in my demands and that my team regarded me as stingy with praise and edgy with criticism. I tell you I trust Donna, so what she said made me feel even worse. I used to be the guy everybody wanted to work for. See, at work as at home, I seem to be losing it."

I then asked Jake about his physical activity. He reported that while he used to play a couple of rounds of golf or tennis on the weekend, and also coach a girl's soccer team, he had stopped doing almost everything over the last several months. "I am just too tired," he responded. "Heck, Dr. Randolph, I know this sounds pathetic but sitting on the sofa and lifting a beer and some chips is about all the exercise I seem to be getting these days. Even that doesn't last very long. I am usually asleep by 8:30 pm. I can't even believe it myself. I mean, I was the biggest Jay Leno fan."

I explained to Jake that many of his presenting complaints and issues could actually be indicators of a change in hormone levels. Jake was quite skeptical that something he could not even see, or had even known to be concerned about, could actually be an underlying cause of the decline in his physical, emotional, and mental health. Still, he said that "Pat would kill me if I didn't let you test out this theory," so he agreed to do a saliva test. His results were as follows:

Hormone Tested	Within Normal Limits (WNL)	Deficiency (DEF)	Excess (EX)
Estrogen: -Estradiol			✔
-Estriol			✔
-Estrone			✔
Progesterone		✔	
Testosterone		✔	

The PSA titer had a result of 1.5 which ruled out prostrate cancer as an imminent diagnosis. In addition, the digital rectal exam was negative for masses. The test results identified hormone imbalance as the causative factor for Jake's presenting symptoms.

I shared the test results with Jake and, then, described for him how I would design a hormonal regimen specific to his needs. Specifically, I told Jake that we needed to address both his condition of estrogen dominance as well as his deficiencies in both progesterone and testosterone. I prescribed for him both testosterone gel and progesterone cream. In addition, I recommended that he take Calcium-D-Glucarate twice daily. As discussed in Chapter 8, this supplement causes excess estrogen to be excreted through the colon.

I then asked Jake to schedule a follow up appointment with me in three months. He abashedly asked if, when he came back, he could again come through the back door. I assured him that my staff would take care of that for him.

Three months later, my nurse came to tell me that somehow our office must have screwed up. Jake was sitting in my waiting room surrounded by about seven other women. She said that, when his appointment was confirmed, nothing was said about the back door and so our scheduler had not known to make any special arrangement about the back door. I asked her to go ahead and bring Jake back.

When I walked into the consultation room, I expected Jake to be upset that we had somehow dropped the ball on protecting his special request for privacy. Instead, Jake stood up and enthusiastically pumped my hand. "Dr. Randolph," he said, "I feel great. I am my old self again and I didn't even need to take one of those little blue pills! Just as you told me, my body had slowed down producing as much of those hormones it needed and I just needed a natural jump start to get me back to where I was before. I am sorry I doubted you."

Jake went on to tell me that his sex drive was back. "In the last month, Pat and I have made love once or twice almost every day. And I tell you, Dr. Randolph, we 'do it' at all times of the day, not just in the morning. I am ready to go in the afternoon when I get home from work and then again before we go to sleep. Just last week Pat told me that, in 'that department,' I am better than I ever was before. If that is true, I guess you could chalk some of my improved sexual performance off to awareness and gratitude."

Jake then told me that his increased energy was translating to other areas, as well. "I am back to playing tennis two nights a week and golf once on the week end. I have even started getting up and either running or doing weights in the mornings. What's more, I am excited about going to work. I get there around 7 a.m. to have some quiet time to brainstorm on new projects. My team seems to feel that I am there for them again and we are making headway on some tight deadlines by all rolling up our sleeves together."

Jake had weighed in 20 lbs. less than when he first came to see me. He said that he had lost the weight without really trying. "I guess you could say that my diet and exercise plan has consisted of moving my bum off the sofa," he commented.

I told Jake that we would do another saliva test to measure his change in hormone levels that day. I also suggested that he return every six months so we could monitor how he was doing and tweak his hormone regimen as needed. "Jake," I said, "I am sorry that my staff forgot to honor your request to come in the back door today, but I assure you that we will handle that better in the future."

Jake responded, "Hey, Doc, that wasn't your staff's fault. I mean, after I found out that I wasn't dying and that my manhood wasn't lost to me forever, I wasn't embarrassed to tell everyone I knew about my hormone imbalance and how you were treating it. I thought, with what you have done for me, the least I could do is sit out there in your waiting room and chat with a few of your patients."

"Think about it, Dr. Randolph," Jake went on, "one of those women could be just like my wife Pat was six months ago. She might have a husband at home who is turning into a bump on a log and she doesn't know why. Even worse, she might think that he doesn't want to or can't get 'it' up because she no longer turns him on. More women and men need to know that male menopause - or andropause, as you called it - is a real thing."

"They also need to know that what goes on with a man's hormones as he ages has more to do with his quality of life than just his ego's need to sexually perform on command. Take me. I felt like I was numbing out to all the good things in my life: my wife, my kids, my work, the activities that I used to enjoy. Now I am back and it didn't take a miracle, years of therapy or a younger wife. It took you telling me what was wrong, and then helping replace the hormones that my body was missing."

"Dr. Randoph, I know now that male menopause is real, but it is not something to fear. There is help. You have shown me that, and maybe if I am willing to talk about it, a few more will know. Tell your staff that when I come back, they can just look for me out front. Maybe by then, I will have a few more men to keep me company. Hey, you might even consider adding *Esquire* and *Field and Stream* to the magazines you order." Jake laughed, "I mean, no offense, but I certainly don't want to get so many new hormones cruising through my body that I start picking up *Redbook* and *Vogue*."

Saliva Testing for Male Hormone Imbalance

Two or more symptoms are an indication of the need to test both Estradiol (E2) and Progesterone. *Source: ZRT Laboratories.*

Hot flashes	Foggy thinking	Depressed
Prostate problems	Increased urinary urge	Sleep disturbances
Headaches	Irritable	Weight gain - hips
Night sweats	Bone loss	Apathy
Decreased urine flow	Nervous	Fatigue
Decreased libido	Anxious	

For two or more symptoms, Testosterone and DHEAS testing is recommended. *Source: ZRT Laboratories.*

Decreased libido	Aches and pains	Heart palpitations
Increased joint pain	Bone loss	Decreased stamina
Increased urinary urge	Oily skin	Anxious
Decreased erections	Foggy thinking	Prostate problems
Depressed	Decrease muscle mass	Decreased urine flow
Burned out feeling	Aggression	Nervous
Fatigue	Decreased flexibility	Decreased mental
Sleep disturbances	Thinning skin	sharpness
Acne	Irritable	

Chapter 13
Human-Identical Hormone Therapy: A Medical Revolution

As the WHI study began to illuminate that synthetic hormone therapies could have significant negative and even life-threatening side effects, the findings ignited feelings of alarm, concern, and fear for both the general public and the medical community. Well-intentioned physicians who had previously relied on synthetic hormones as the treatment of choice for their patients suffering from symptoms associated with peri-menopause and menopause were suddenly confused and stymied. Female patients who used to clamor for anything that would relieve them from the hot flashes, night sweats, insomnia, mood swings, and many other unpleasant symptoms associated with hormonal imbalance shifted their attitudes. The media has reported how the WHI study found a link between synthetic hormones and cancer, stroke, and Alzheimer's, and women have begun both to challenge their physicians while also taking the initiative to research safer and more natural alternatives.

Watch Out! Here Comes The Informed Healthcare Consumer

A key trend affecting women's healthcare providers today is that female consumers are agents of change. They demand that their physicians and other care providers evidence a mastery of knowledge. These informed healthcare consumers are looking to the medical community to provide them with information, choice, convenience, and a more comprehensive approach to health and wellness.

In her book, *Market Driven Healthcare: Who Wins, Who Loses in the Transformation of America's Largest Service Industry*, Rita Herzlinger states:

"Many of today's middle-aged female baby boomers are consumer revolutionaries, as they are the highest-earning and most educated group of women ever, as well as the fastest-growing segment of the women's market."

In years past, women and men simply relied on their doctors to decide what was wrong with them, and then to tell them what to do. A decade ago, patient interaction was typically a one-way monologue where a physician's diagnosis and treatment recommendations were most often accepted without question. Those days are over.

Today, a physician's conversation with a patient is much different and, I believe, the change is for the better. Patients ask questions, challenge medical opinions and seek out medical second opinions. In my own practice, I find that more and more of my patients want me to supply them with information and data so that they can make informed choices; however, they don't just rely on me to feed them what I think they should know. Women walk into my office armed with research they have pulled off the internet and notes they have made while watching health specials on television. They go to the library to research topics and get on internet chat boards to learn from others' experiences with similar health issues.

As a physician, I recognize that my role has shifted dramatically over the last several years. I am no longer the "all-knowing one." When my patients value and respect my medical opinion, we then engage in an active dialogue. Today I am privileged to serve as a key member of my patient's "health team."

In the aftermath of the WHI study, more and more women want alternatives when it comes to hormone replacement. When their physicians can't help them evaluate what else is out there, they search it out for themselves. Many women who previously took synthetic hormones because their physicians prescribed them are now bitter and angry. They feel that the traditional medical community sold them short and put them at risk.

 Because of the dangers of synthetic hormone replacement, the option of human-identical hormone therapy has recently become a hot topic. As I mentioned in the Introduction, hormone therapy is a frequent talk show topic. Dr. Phil and his wife Robin McGraw have actually hosted a series entitled "Hormones From Hell" in which Robin shared her own personal experience using a combination of human-identical hormone therapy and natural supplements to ease menopausal symptoms.

Early in 2004, the actress and author Suzanne Somers released her new book *The Sexy Years: Discover The Hormone Connection*. Many of my physician peers were astounded that Ms. Somers's book quickly rose to the top of the New York Times bestseller list and that many of their patients walked into their offices with a highlighted copy in hand. They ask me, "How can patients turn to and trust media personalities when it comes to medical information?"

I simply reply, "As a physician, I am more sad that our medical community and the pharmaceutical industry have given women reasons not to trust us. I think that if we physicians look at this changing paradigm with an open attitude, we have the opportunity to move into and participate in an exciting revolution occurring right now in the healthcare industry. As physicians, we are all trained to be patient advocates. Should it not be our mission to be on the leading edge of exploring and understanding both conventional therapies as well as non-pharmaceutical treatments that may be safer and more efficacious for our patients?"

In most cases, my physician colleagues pause for a moment to reflect on how this new era of consumer-driven medicine will change their role. Then, with varying degrees of skepticism, acceptance, resistance, and/or reticence, they acknowledge that perhaps there is some merit in a medical model where the patient plays an active instead of a passive role and where traditional medical thinking and training are challenged rather than automatically endorsed. Over the last couple of years, I have seen many physicians gradually embrace the transformation of the old medical model. Most of them report to me that, after a while, they find that this "new consumer-driven model of healthcare" creates new and exciting opportunities for learning and interaction.

As these physicians change their mindsets regarding patient/consumer roles, they also change their approaches to hormone therapy replacement. The skepticism they may have previously had regarding human-identical hormone therapies is replaced with amazement once they listen to their patients' positive reports and personally witness the undeniable clinical manifestations associated with hormonal balancing.

One colleague I had previously regarded as stodgy and unreachable because he had been openly derisive about my practice of prescribing and compounding human-identical hormone therapies stopped me outside the operating room not long ago. "Randy," he said, "I had steadfastly refused to try those 'natural' (human-identical) hormones you've been so vehement about until I had a patient point-blank ask me: why would I continue to prescribe synthetic hormones when I knew that they could be putting my patients at risk if there was an alternative that posed no risk at all? I tried to explain away her concerns and even pooh-poohed what I called a 'flower-child' movement away from tried and true pharmaceuticals. Well, I tell you, that woman got up and stalked out of my office. In over thirty years of practice, that had never happened before. I am a physician but I am also a businessman. Her leaving without looking back sure got my attention."

"Over the next several months, I listened a lot more closely when my patients asked me about alternatives to synthetic hormones. I really heard their concerns about taking something that they had read had many unsafe side effects. I also felt more compassion than I ever had before when my patients talked about how their menopausal symptoms often made their lives so miserable that the idea of not taking anything at all to help seemed like a death sentence."

He continued, "I realized that I needed to educate myself, so I started reading all the research I could get my hands on about alternative treatments. I was surprised at the substance of the clinical evidence in favor of human-identical hormone replacement. I have to tell you that I actually advised several of my patients who were adamant about coming off their synthetic treatment to go down to your Natural Medicine Shoppe and just try some of your over-the-counter progesterone cream. Nine out of ten times, that was all they needed to get symptomatic relief. From what I have learned, I am sure that the tenth patient probably needs more than just human-identical progesterone."

He looked me straight in the eye as he said, "I don't feel comfortable yet interpreting a saliva test and then writing a prescription for an individualized compound of human-identical hormones. Would you be willing to consult with me on this case?"

Of course, my answer was affirmative. As I walked on, I realized that I had just witnessed a true example of consumer-driven healthcare. One patient had had the power to ask for what she wanted and, in the process, start a domino effect that changed one physician's practice patterns forever.

Today's Woman Has Mind, Body, and Spirit

I believe that women are exquisitely complex. It has been my experience that my female patients are often much more aware than their male counterparts about how their thoughts, feelings, and physiology interact to define their health. In this view, health is not just a matter of feeling well enough to go to work, make dinner, or go to an aerobics class. Rather, health is determined by an interaction among genetics, environment, and lifestyle situations. Most women recognize that their stress, lifestyle, attitudes, behaviors, supportive relationships, economic well-being, access to healthcare, as well as a sense of spiritual purpose can all contribute to or subtract from their condition of health.

To treat women today, I believe physicians and the entire medical community must commit energies to developing a medical model that supports a woman's need to be whole and complete in mind, body, emotion, and spirit. Herbert Benson, M.D., and his colleagues at Harvard Medical School were among the first to verify the potency of the mind-body-spirit connection. Their work with the relaxation response has led to a cascade of findings about how mind/body mechanisms can be used for medically significant impact on hypertension, heart disease, cancer, and other conditions.

As a gynecologist who has treated tens of thousands of women with hormone imbalances, I always engage my patients in a discussion about their lifestyle issues, situational stresses, and feelings of fulfillment or lack of fulfillment. I am very clear that I am not equipped to be a therapist, but that I am available to be a good listener. I must say that it is rare for me to interact with a patient who doesn't report some feelings of stress or a sense of being overwhelmed.

I see that my primary job is to identify and treat any underlying hormonal imbalance that can be causing or contributing to mental and/or emotional dysfunction. Saliva testing provides me with the diagnostic data I need to prescribe a medically sound and precise hormone replacement regimen for each individual patient. Still, I know that while human-identical hormone replacement works on a cellular level to promote health and well-being, it is still a single-faceted approach to treating a multi-faceted being. When I look at the big picture of all the factors influencing health, I can see that many of the mental, emotional, and spiritual forces are within the direct control of the individual.

When my patients share with me that they feel pulled in too many directions, I frequently encourage them to experiment with different techniques to help with relaxation and meditation. Meditation has been shown to reduce stress, panic, anxiety, and pain. It has also been shown to reduce muscle tension and decrease blood pressure. Hot flashes cause a reaction similar to a stress response and relaxation techniques may therefore help reduce hot flashes.

As a practice, yoga integrates breathing exercises, physical postures, and meditation. I have practiced yoga off and on over the years, and I have many patients who are committed to their yoga practice. Benefits of yoga have been found to include increases in muscle strength, muscle mass, a sense of peacefulness, and increased vigor. Yoga students frequently report decreases in anxiety, depression, and fatigue.

Exercise also has many health benefits beyond just improving body shape and accelerating weight loss. My bottom line is: *Move more* and you will *feel better*. Many of my patients tell me that walking or running every day gives them both personal space and a physical work out. Weight bearing exercises also have great merit, including helping to build bone mass and increasing mental focus. Swimming is an excellent all over exercise that doesn't put stress on the joints. Dancing or aerobics can contribute to cardiovascular health while also convening a community for fun and social interactions. My advice: Whatever you do to *exercise*, do it *regularly* and *joyfully*.

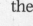 The use of mind/body techniques occurs within a broader context when it comes to choosing or changing a lifestyle to promote health. Making a daily practice of mind/body techniques and exercise are but two of several areas of lifestyle change that work together in a synergistic way. Other areas can include social support and spiritual consciousness.

While the benefits of diet and exercise are obvious, there is a growing body of research indicating that supportive interpersonal relationships are strongly associated with better health. They seem to ameliorate or buffer the harmful effects of stress on the body. I have found that women who are going through "the change of life" feel better about themselves and their personal metamorphosis when they are in some form of community with other like-minded women. The sense of emotional sharing and validation that women can give to one another can't be found in a pill.

Women tell me that when they can openly discuss their physical, mental, and emotional changes with their male partners they struggle less with self-esteem issues typically associated with menopause and aging. Men who make the time to listen, comfort, encourage, pick up take out dinners, and occasionally give unsolicited back rubs to a hassled wife/girlfriend/lover/sister can provide an invaluable source of social support within the walls of a woman's own home. If anyone could patent a formula for an empathetic mate, I have no doubt that baby-boomer women would catapult that person to fame and fortune overnight.

While the idea of mind/body medicine may not seem that far-fetched, you may be wondering what I mean by "Spirit." I do have a very strong personal belief in a Higher Power but, in this context, my intention is not to preach or convert. I will say, however, that I believe that every person's feeling of health and well-being is enhanced when they are able to connect to something larger than themselves.

I often talk with people who truly believe that they can control their world. This need to be in control is frequently accompanied by feelings of tension and stress. These people believe that they must face the world alone. I see that their hyper-independence and self-imposed isolation too often fosters physical manifestations and symptoms of poor health.

In contrast, I find that people who at some level espouse or experience a feeling of interdependence with something beyond themselves have within them an antidote to the effects of stress. Whatever "Spirit" may mean for these people, studies have shown that people with this mindset experience enhanced effectiveness of the body's immune defenses and more zealous self-repair mechanisms. For some people this "Spirit" connection happens through a religious experience, for others it occurs when they walk alongside an ocean, hear a child laugh, or observe a planted seed transform into a tomato bush.

Why do I bring up the importance of a "Spirit" connection? Remember, hormonal changes usher in lifecycle changes. A child becomes a young woman who can reproduce; a mother becomes a wise woman holding her power in new ways; a grandmother moves from serving as primary caretaker to overseeing the ebb and flow of her clan. I have found that a woman who is attuned with her "Spirit" is better able to flow more gracefully and peacefully into the new roles that have been hormonally scripted for her life.

A New Era of Medicine: Relationship-Centered Care

Most physicians and health care providers today are reeling from how managed care has impacted their practice and approach to patient care. The hard truth is that managed care has been an economic strategy developed to restrain the healthcare costs associated with treating sick people. To date, the payors, e.g. the government and the insurance companies, have spent very little substantive effort to build a model where preventive care is rewarded and the intrinsic benefits of patient advocacy are supported.

The business reality for physicians today is that they need to see more patients in less time. This does not lend itself to a caring, responsive interaction where there is time to listen and probe beyond the surface of a patient's presenting symptoms. Physicians and patients too often find themselves caught in a vise where patients feel like they are just "a number" and physicians feel pressed to know more about insurance billing codes than they know about the life stresses and joys of their patients. This scenario of dollars driving patient care is an affront. I believe it is time for all of us to do what we can to rebel against the mechanization of the healing industry.

Is it possible to stay in business as a healthcare provider and also deliver healthcare services in a personalized and caring environment? I believe that it is, but doing so is certainly not easy. Physicians, like myself, who have in their hearts a commitment to offering a relationship-centered approach to service must remember that healthcare always begins with an intimate one-on-one interaction. Pain, disease, and discomfort are personal. Lifecycle changes can be frightening. Family dynamics and professional stresses play dominant roles in health and well-being.

I certainly don't have all the answers, but I do have a very personal commitment to the Hippocratic Oath. I believe that I have to take responsibility for finding the ways and means to ensure that my role as a patient advocate remains my top priority. In a stringent managed care environment, this isn't easy, and I don't always succeed. Still, here are a few very basic philosophies I strive to enact everyday:

- **Listen, listen, listen**: Try to respect patients as individuals and honor their experiences as valid. Challenge yourself everyday to open up ears of compassion to explore beyond the physical realm to best understand how a person's life experiences are entwined to define their state of health, disease, or healing.

- **Educate, facilitate, participate**: An individual's lifestyle choices largely determine their state of health and well-being. First, take the time to educate patients regarding underlying causative factors related to their presenting concern as well as options/alternatives for treatment. Then, firmly place control for healthcare decisions in their hands. As a physician, I believe my role should be to facilitate knowledge transfer before participating in patient care, treatment, and recovery.

- **Learn, improve, expand**: For every physician practicing in today's managed care environment, time is the most precious commodity. Still, if possible, I recommend dedicating two to three weeks a year to attending medical education programs that provide information on new treatment modalities and integrative models of care. Remain open-minded and receptive to innovation and experimentation, but analyze all new ideas with the scientific discipline of thought characteristic of medical school training.

- **Remain fiscally responsible**: Accept and acknowledge that physicians are healthcare providers who are also in the *business of delivering healthcare services.* Wisely use economic resources to support business solvency. If a medical practice is not solvent, the physician won't be around to be a patient advocate. In other words, no margin = no mission.

- **Start now**: Don't wait for the healthcare environment in which you practice to change. Be responsible for creating a microcosm of relationship-centered care with each patient encounter. Believe that you can become the image of your highest values.

If you are a patient or informed healthcare consumer, you too have to take responsibility for transforming today's seemingly sterile and financially-focused healthcare delivery system into one that inspires and promotes trusting and responsible relationships between the caregiver and the recipient. As an individual or family-member, I encourage you to make the effort to step up to the plate. Here are a few of things you can do:

- **Learn, learn, learn**: Take responsibility for educating yourself regarding both health, illness, and treatment options. Don't be afraid to peek outside the box of conventional medical thinking, but find and analyze the scientific data that supports any "healing" claims associated with alternative products or treatment modalities.

- **Question, dialogue, challenge**: Recognize that as a person/patient, you are the ultimate informed decision maker. Ask your doctors questions, dialogue with them about options and alternatives, challenge their opinions when appropriate. Get second opinions. Find your voice and speak your mind. Don't give up your power as you move forward to find common ground regarding next steps.

- **Share, connect, partner**: Illness and disease can be frightening. Change of life symptoms can be overwhelming. Learning that you are not alone can be very helpful. Find ways to connect with others with the same concern. Learn and grow from their stories and experiences.

- **Make healthy choices**: Incorporate prevention and health awareness into every day. Because our society moves so fast, most people don't think about their health until they are sick. Become more aware of how important all the lifestyle decisions you make several times a day really are. You do not have to be a victim. Make healthy choices about nutrition, exercise, meditation and relaxation, social support, environments, and habits.

- **Embrace your whole self**: Your mind, body, emotions, and spirit all play a role in defining your uniqueness and your health. Regard your body as a sanctuary while you also attend to and respect the less visible but no less potent facets of who you are. Do not devalue the importance of feelings and intuition.

- **Be realistic**: No one likes being sick. I haven't seen any active baby-boomer men or women standing in line to experience the first health maladies associated with aging. In addition, I have yet to meet a woman who is excited about experiencing symptoms associated with hormonal shifts and imbalances. I believe that medical miracles and spontaneous healing really can happen, but in most cases, healing and renewed commitment to health takes time to manifest. I find that patients who are best able to sustain a feeling of health and well-being understand the importance of participating and nurturing the healing process.

In summary, we are now moving into an era where buzzwords like "integrative medicine" and "mind-body-spirit-care" are frequently and loosely bandied about. We must not allow these philosophies to be weakened until they are nothing more than marketing ploys. We - physicians, healthcare providers, informed healthcare consumers - have the power to enliven an approach to healthcare delivery that blends state-of-the-art conventional medicine with complementary or alternative approaches, while also incorporating an openness to a spiritual dimension of care.

Relationship-centered care means that patients are involved and informed in any decision impacting their care, treatment, or healing. The informed healthcare consumer has a voice and participates rather than passively waiting for advice and following directives. The time is now to implement an interactive healthcare model. If we all do our part, I believe that we have the power to mitigate some of the depersonalization inherent in the current managed care environment, and in the process, I think we may redefine "health" and reap some surprising benefits.

Chapter 14

Resource Listing: Getting Help When and Where You Need It

Okay, so what now? Let's say that you are a physician or healthcare consumer and you've just finished this book. You have read about the advantages and benefits of human-identical hormone therapies but you may still be skeptical. Or you may have all the data you need to move forward for first hand experience with whether or not human-identical hormone therapies offer a more safe and effective alternative to synthetic HRT. Regardless, where do you go from here?

The goal of this chapter is to provide you with a list of resources that can help you further your education regarding human-identical hormone replacement and/or move forward immediately to take action. I am including information that should help you: (1) find/access a healthcare professional to guide you through your diagnostic and treatment regimen, (2) find a source for individualized prescriptions, and (3) identify options for purchasing over-the-counter human-identical progesterone products.

Please note: the contact information listed in this section is current as of the publication of this book.

The Natural Hormone Institute of America

In bringing the dream of this book to life, I realized just how great the need is to continue sharing information and championing the cause of human-identical hormone therapies as a safe and effective alternative to synthetic HRT. As a result, I founded The Natural Hormone Institute of America in 2003 with two goals in mind. My first goal is to provide a framework for my mission to educate both the medical community and the healthcare consumer about human-identical hormone therapies. My second goal is to create a business structure that will promote more widespread use of human-identical hormone products and prescriptions, while also fostering ongoing research in the burgeoning field of hormone replacement. Since the Institute's founding, I have been overwhelmed by the positive responses of many of my physician peers, as well as by interested and educated healthcare consumers. I am grateful that The Natural Hormone Institute of America appears to be meeting a very real need at a crucial time.

For more information regarding human-identical hormone replacement, to discuss scheduling a personal consultation, or for specific product information about my signature over-the-counter progesterone cream, please direct your queries to:

Genie James, M.M.Sc., Executive Director
The Natural Hormone Institute of America
1891 Beach Boulevard Suite 300
Jacksonville Beach, Florida 32250
Phone: 866-628-6337
Website: http://www.safesthormones.com

Compounding Pharmacies

Throughout this book, I'm sure you have noticed a recurring theme that "one-size-does-NOT-fit-all" when it comes to hormone replacement. As you learned in Chapter 5, compounding pharmacies can be a resource for physicians who are interested in moving away from the use of synthetic

HRT, but do not have the experience or training in new areas such as the use of saliva testing, and the subsequent prescription of human-identical hormones. Today's compounding pharmacies can produce literally whatever the doctor orders. This means that a physician can work with a compounding pharmacy to develop personalized prescriptions of human-identical hormones to meet the unique needs of each individual patient.

If you have never before heard, or used a compounding pharmacy, here are some key facts that you may want to consider:

- Every compounding pharmacy is licensed and inspected by the State Pharmacy Board.

- Compounding pharmacists are educated and trained to provide information regarding the formulation of human-identical hormones; they can reassure, educate, and provide physicians with safe dosage guidelines for human-identical hormone supplementation.

- All materials used in compounding formulations are subject to FDA inspection and the agency's Good Manufacturing Procedures code.

While I have my own compounding pharmacy as a part of my practice, there are two compounding pharmacies that I often recommend to other physicians. They are listed on the next page.

1. College Pharmacy. Phone: 800-888-9358.
   3505 Austin Bluffs Parkway, Suite 101
   Colorado Springs, CO 80918
   Website: http://www.collegepharmacy.com

2. Women's International Pharmacy.
   Phone: 800-279-5708.
   2 Marsh Court
   Madison, WI 53718
   Website: http://www.womensinternational.com

In addition, there are many other credible compounding pharmacies across the United States. To locate a pharmacy that provides individualized prescriptions, contact:

The International Academy of Compounding Pharmacists (IACP)

P.O. Box 1365

Sugar Land, TX 7787

Phone: 281-933-8400

Fax: 281-495-0602

Website: http://www.iacprx.org

Background: IACP was established in 1991 as Professionals and Patients for Customized Care (P2C2). In 1996, P2C2 changed its name to IACP in an effort to broaden its scope and recognize changes in the profession. Today, the IACP has more than 1,800 members internationally, serving pharmacists, physicians, students, and patients.

Professional Compounding Centers of America (PCCA)
9901 South Wilcrest Drive
Houston, TX 77099
Phone: 877-798-3224
Fax: 877-765-1422
Website: http://www.pccarx.com

Background: PCCA provides independent pharmacists with a complete support system for compounding unique dosage forms. Founded in 1981, PCCA has more than 3,000 pharmacist members located throughout the United States, Canada, Australia, Europe, and New Zealand. On average, PCCA's consulting department answers more than 500 calls a day, providing members with comprehensive technical support.

Over-The-Counter Human-Identical Progesterone Creams

As a woman enters her mid-thirties and until she is in her late forties, she can be said to be pre-menopausal. A woman in this lifecycle is in her middle reproductive years. It is during these years that the balance of hormones produced by the endocrine system first begins to shift. As you have learned, progesterone, the "feel good" hormone, is the first hormone to decline and drops 120 times more rapidly than estrogen.

As progesterone begins to decline and estrogen becomes the dominant hormone within a woman's system, symptoms such as PMS, breast swelling, irregular periods, fluid retention, uterine fibroids, reduced libido and migraine headaches can occur. From their mid-thirties on, almost all women are estrogen dominant.

In many cases, this condition of estrogen dominance can be neutralized by administering over-the-counter transdermal human-identical progesterone cream. Once the body's optimum hormonal ratio of estrogen to progesterone is restored, most unpleasant symptoms will be eliminated.

You can buy some form of "natural" progesterone cream over-the-counter in most health food stores. The good news is that it is available. The bad news is that you don't always know what you are getting. Most of the product labels do not specify whether or not they meet the following criteria for product excellence. Key questions to ask before purchasing any progesterone product:

- Is the progesterone truly human-identical?
- Is the concentration appropriate for you?
- Do the hormones used in the formulation meet the United States Pharmacopoeia gold standards for quality and purity?
- Was the progesterone product actually compounded under the strict guidelines approved by the National Association of Compounding Pharmacists?
- Is the concentration of oil in the cream formulation one that will promote or inhibit transdermal absorption?

The following are progesterone creams that I have reviewed and am confident that they contain human-identical progesterone:

C. W. Randolph, Jr., M.D.
Dr. C. W. Randolph's Natural Progesterone Cream
1891 Beach Blvd. Suite 200
Jacksonville Beach, Florida 32250
(866) 628-6337 or www.safesthormones.com

Arbonne International
PhytoProlief and Prolief Natural Balancing Creams
P.O. Box 2488
Laguna Hills, California
(800) ARBONNE or www.arbonne.com

Emerita
Pro-Gest progesterone cream
621 SW Alder, Suite 900
Portland, Oregon 97205-3627
(800) 648-8211 or www.progest.com

The Health and Science Research Institute
Serenity for Women progesterone cream
661 Beville Rd., Suite 101
Daytona Beach, Florida 32119
(888) 222-1415 or www.health-science.com

HM Enterprises
Happy PMS
2622 Bailey Drive
Norcross, Georgia 30071
(800) 742-4773 or www.hmenterprises.com

Life-flo Health Care Products
Progestacare Cream
8146 N. 23rd Ave, Suite E
Phoenix, Arizona 85021
(888) 999-7440 or www.shield.com/lifeflo

Products of Nature
Natural Woman progesterone cream
54 Danbury Road
Ridgefield, Connecticut 06877
(800) 665-5952 or www.pronature.com

Restored Balance, Inc.
Restored Balance PMS/Menopausal progesterone cream
42 Meadowbridge Dr., SW
Cartersville, Georgia
(800) 865-7499 or www.restoredbalanceusa.com

There are many other progesterone creams on the market today that I have not reviewed which may also contain human-identical progesterone. If you have any doubt or concerns regarding any human-identical progesterone product call the company and ask how many milligrams of progesterone per ounce the cream contains.

When an over-the-counter human-identical progesterone cream does not completely eliminate unpleasant symptoms, this can be regarded as a signal that a woman's estrogen and/or testosterone levels have also begun to decline. At this time, a saliva test is an appropriate next step to determine the current ratio of all three sex hormones.

Saliva Testing of Hormones

A complete and individualized hormone profile is needed to provide a rational basis for correcting any hormone imbalance. To date, saliva testing has been found to be the most accurate tool for testing the spectrum of hormone activity and levels. Saliva testing is the most reliable way to measure free, "bioavailable," hormone activity; e.g. the hormones that are actually available to do their job at the cellular level. Because hormones bind to the carrier proteins in blood serum, blood tests do not effectively measure amounts of bioavailable hormone levels. Similarly, while urine testing can give a reading of "good" estrogen levels versus "bad" estrogen levels, it does not provide an accurate reading of other hormone activity, such as levels of progesterone or testosterone.

Saliva testing can quickly and easily illuminate the interaction of estrogen, progesterone, testosterone, cortisol, and DHEA levels. Because each hormone plays a vital role in maintaining the body's optimum function, knowledge of an imbalance in one or more of these hormones can help identify the underlying cause of many health concerns.

Here are a few other facts for anyone considering adding saliva testing into their diagnostic regimen:

- Saliva testing is painless; no needles

- Saliva collection is easy and convenient

- Saliva can be preserved for up to one month to allow

for additional testing if needed.

One of my personal mentors, Dr. David Zava, developed saliva testing as a simple non-invasive means to identify hormone imbalances associated with diminished health and well-being. Over the past 25 years, Dr. Zava has built on his skills as a biochemist and research scientist to publish more than 60 clinical research papers on the effects of estrogen and progesterone on breast cancer. He is also the co-author with John R. Lee, M.D. of *What Your Doctor May Not Tell You About Breast Cancer: How Hormone Balance Can Help Save Your Life.*

In 1998, Dr. Zava established ZRT Laboratory. I use ZRT Laboratory and recommend it to others because:

- ZRT Laboratory is the only large-volume clinical laboratory to extract saliva to remove contaminants that can alter test results. Other commercial labs use straight saliva and do not extract interfering factors.

- ZRT Laboratory is one of the few labs to carefully monitor and report hormone type, dosage, and timing.

- ZRT Laboratory is the only laboratory that monitors and reports symptoms and relates them to hormone test results.

- ZRT Laboratory's staff of credentialed physicians and trained personnel offers education and training, as well as assistance with interpreting test results.

To initiate a relationship or to find out more information, contact:

ZRT Laboratories
1815 NW 169th Place, Suite 5050
Beaverton, OR 97006
Phone: 503-466-2445
FAX: 503-466-1636
Website: http://www.salivatest.com

Biopharmaceutical Companies

As I stated at the conclusion of Chapter 3, I am grateful to report that today there are several specialty biopharmaceutical companies dedicating resources and dollars to developing proprietary human-identical/bio-identical hormone products. The following is a list of some of the products with which I am currently familiar and prescribe in my own practice. Each of these has been approved by the FDA.

Human-Identical Estradiol
Brand name: **Estrasorb**
Mode of Delivery: Topical emulsion/transdermal
                        application
Manufacturer: Novavax, Inc.
Marketed by: Novavax, Inc. Corporate Headquarters
            8320 Guilford Road, Suite C
            Columbia, Maryland 21046
            www.novavax.com

Brand name: **EstroGel**
Mode of Delivery: Topical emulsion/transdermal
application
Manufacturer: R. P. Scherger North America
Marketed by: Solvay Pharmaceuticals, Inc. Corporate
Headquarters
Marietta, Georgia 30062
www.solvaypharmaceuticals.com

Brand name: **Estrace**
Mode of Delivery: Estradiol tablets/oral adminstration
Manufacturer: Bristol-Myers Squibb Co.
Marketed by: Warner Chilcott, Inc.
Rockaway, NJ 07866
www.estrace.com

There are also many generic forms of estradiol on the
market, as well as many estradiol skin "patches" currently
available by prescription from a physician. It is also important
to note that the product inserts for most of these products
state that: "using human-identical estrodiol products without
human-identical progesterone may increase the risk of heart
attacks, strokes, breast cancer and blood clots."

Human-Identical Progesterone
Brand name: **Crinone**
Mode of Delivery: Bioadhesive vaginal gel
Manufacturer: Serono, Inc.
Marketed by: Serono, Inc. Corporate Headquarters
One Technology Place
Rockland, Maryland 02370

www.seronousa.com

Brand name: **Prochieve**

Mode of Delivery: Bioadhesive vaginal gel

Manufacturer: Columbia Laboratories, Inc.

Marketed by: Columbia Laboratories, Inc.
354 Eisenhower Parkway
Second Floor, Plaza 1
Livingston, New Jersey 07039
www.columbialabs.com

Brand name: **Prometrium**

Mode of Delivery: Micronized progesterone in peanut oil/
capsules/oral administration

Manufacturer: R. P. Scherger North America

Marketed by: Solvay Pharmaceuticals, Inc. Corporate
Headquarters
Marietta, Georgia 30062
www.solvaypharmaceuticals.com

Human-Identical Testosterone

Brand name: **Androgel**

Mode of Delivery: Testosterone gel/transdermal application

Marketed by: Solvay Pharmaceuticals, Inc. Corporate
Headquarters
Marietta, Georgia 30062
www.androgel.com

Brand name: **Testoderm**

Mode of Delivery: Skin patch

Manufacturer: ALZA Corporation

Marketed by: 1900 Charleston Road
Mountain View, California 94043
www.alza.com

Physician Opportunities

Over the last several years, many of my physician peers have contacted me with an interest in learning more about my practice model. They want to know more about my dispensing component for human-identical hormone therapies and a Natural Medicine Shoppe offering complementary/natural medicine products to my patients. In early 2004, I made the decision to co-found a company - LIVESSE, LLC - that could effectively respond to these physicians and support them in their efforts to expand their practice delivery model. Today, LIVESSE, LLC brings to physicians a franchising opportunity for adding natural/complementary medicine and human-identical hormone products into a medical practice. For more information, contact:

Rick Buchsbaum, CEO
LIVESSE, LLC
109 Westpark Drive, Suite 150
Brentwood, Tennessee 37027
Phone: 866-454-8377
http://www.livesse.com

Want to Know More? Recommended Reading

As I have mentioned throughout the book, there are many other physician pioneers who have helped lay a foundation of learning and knowledge in the study of human-identical hormone therapy. I have the following books in my personal library. Each author offers the reader the benefit of additional information and another perspective. Please note that these resources are not prioritized by perceived merit but are listed in alphabetical order according to author.

Lee, John R., M.D., *Natural Progesterone, The Multiple Role Of A Remarkable Hormone.* Sebastopol, California: BLL Publishing, 1993.

Lee, John R., M.D., with Virginia Hopkins. *What Your Doctor May Not Tell You About Menopause.* New York: Warner Books, 1996.

Lee, John R., M.D., with Jesse Hanley, M.D., and Virginia Hopkins. *What Your Doctor May Not Tell You About Perimenopause.* New York: Warner Books, 1999.

Lee, John R., M.D., with David Zava, Ph.D., and Virginia Hopkins. *What Your Doctor May Not Tell You About Breast Cancer. How Hormone Balance Can Help Save Your Life.* New York: Warner Books, 2002.

Northrup, Christiane, M.D., *Women's Bodies, Women's Wisdom: Creating Physical and Emotional Health and Healing.* New York: Bantam Books, 1994.

Northrup, Christiane, M.D., *The Wisdom Of Menopause: Creating Physical and Emotional Health and Healing During the Change.* New York: Bantam Books, 2001.

Schwartz, Erika, M.D., *The Hormone Solution.* New York:

Warner Books, 2002.

Shulman, Neil, M.D., and Edmunds, Kim S., M.D., *Healthy Transitions: A Woman's Guide to Perimenopause, Menopause & Beyond.* New York: Prometheus Books, 2004.

Somers, Suzanne, *The Sexy Years, Discover The Hormone Connection: The Secret To Fabulous Sex, Great Health, And Vitality For Women and Men.* New York: Crown Publishers, 2004.

Taylor, Eldred, M.D., and Bell-Taylor, Ava, M.D., *Are Your Hormones Making You Sick?.* Physicians Natural Medicine, Inc., 2000.

Whitaker, Julian, M.D., *Dr. Whitaker's Guide to Natural Hormone Replacement.* Potomac, Maryland: Phillips Publishing, 1999.

Wilson, James L., N.D., D.C., Ph.D., *Adrenal Fatigue.* Petaluma, CA: Smart Publications, 2003.

Wright, Jonathan V., M.D., and John Morgenthaler, *Natural Hormone Replacement For Women Over 45.* Petaluma, CA: Smart Publications, 1997.

The Best Resource: Yourself

As I end this book, I want to take a moment to remind each reader that no one can tell you what is right for you or for your health. I encourage you to listen, read, ask questions and seek out others who feel that they are in "hormone hell" to share information and experiences. I applaud you for seeking additional medical counsel to better understand your options and choices for hormone replacement. Once you have the data in hand, I believe that the most important thing you can do is to get quiet and listen to your heart. Within each of us is the wisdom we need to make the 'right' decisions.

Glossary

2-hydroxyesterone – An estrogen metabolite. The role of 2-hydroxyestrone (2-OHE1) in breast cancer has been the subject of considerable controversy on the issue of whether it is carcinogenic or anticarcinogenic. The current conclusion is that 2-OHE1 is anticarcinogenic.

2-hydroxyestradiol – A metabolite of estradiol, antioxidant and a "good estrogen."

16-hydroxestrone – A metabolite of estradiol, carcinogenic and a "bad estrogen."

Adrenal Exhaustion – When the adrenal glands are not functioning optimally, you can have a condition that is known as adrenal exhaustion. Adrenal fatigue often develops after periods of intense or lengthy physical or emotional stress, when overstimulation of the glands leave them unable to meet your body's needs. Some other names for the syndrome include non-Addison's hypoadrenia, sub-clinical hypoadrenia, hypoadrenalism, and neurasthenia.

Adrenal Gland – A small, triangular-shaped endocrine gland located on the top of each kidney. Each adrenal gland is approximately 3 inches wide, and a half inch high. It produces three groups of cortical hormones (adrenal steroids): mineralocorticoids, glucocorticoids, and gonadocorticoids. Epinephrine and norepinephrine (non-steroids) are also produced.

Adrenal Steroid – The adrenal glands produce three groups of steroids: mineralocorticoids, glucocorticoids and gonadocorticoids. The principal mineralocorticoid is aldosterone, which acts to conserve sodium ions and water in the body. The principal glucocorticoid is cortisol, which increases blood glucose levels. The third group of steroids is the gonadocorticoids, or sex hormones. Female hormones (estrogens) are secreted in minimal amounts by the adrenal cortex, but their effect is usually masked by the hormones from ovaries.

Alzheimer's Disease - The most common form of dementia among older people, Alzheimer's disease involves the parts of the brain that control thought, memory, and language. This brain disorder seriously affects a person's ability to carry out daily activities. Although scientists are learning more every day, right now they still do not know what causes AD, and there is no cure.

Amenorrhea – An absence or abnormal cessation of the menses (menstruation).

Anatomy – The bodily structure of a plant or an animal or any of its parts.

Androgenic Hormones – Also known as androgens. Steroid hormones that stimulate or control the development and maintenance of masculine characteristics and add in the development of male secondary sex characteristics. The primary, and most well known, androgen is testosterone. All natural androgens are steroid derivatives of androstane. They are also the precursor of all estrogens. A subset of androgens, adrenal androgens, includes steroids that function as weak steroids or steroid precursors, including dehydroepiandrosterone (DHEA), dehydroepiandrosterone sulfate (DHEA-S), and androstenedione.

Androgens – See Androgenic Hormones.

Androstenediol – A steroid metabolite.

Androstenedione – An androgenic steroid secreted by the ovaries, adrenal gland and testes. Androstenediones are the parent structure of estrone and are also converted metabolically to testosterone and other androgens.

Atrophy – The reduction of or wasting of tissues, organs, or the entire body as a result of the reabsorption of cells, hormonal changes, diminished cellular proliferation, decreased cellular volume, death.

Bioavailable – The ability of a drug or other substance to be absorbed and used by the body. Distinct from its potency; proportion of the administered dose that is absorbed into the bloodstream.

Biochemistry – The chemistry of living organisms and the chemical, molecular, and physical changes occurring therein.

Bio-Identical - Bio-identical means "exactly the same," "identical" to the molecule produced by the human body.

Blood Clot - Blood clots (fibrin clots) are the clumps that result from coagulation of the blood. A blood clot that forms in a vessel or within the heart and remains there is called a thrombus. A thrombus that travels from the vessel or heart chamber where it formed to another location in the body is called an embolus, and the disorder, an embolism (for example, pulmonary embolism).

Blood Serum – The clear liquid that separates from the blood when it is allowed to clot completely. This watery fluid of the blood contains fibrinogen, a clotting agent.

Bone Mass Density (BMD) - Also called bone mineral density test. Bone mineral density is a measured calculation of the true mass of bone. The absolute amount of bone as measured by bone mineral density (BMD) generally correlates with bone strength and its ability to bear weight. By measuring BMD, it is possible to predict fracture risk in the same manner that measuring blood pressure can help predict the risk of stroke. BMD cannot predict the certainty of developing a fracture; it can only predict risk.

Breast Cancer - Breast cancer is a malignant growth that begins in the tissues of the breast. Any of the types of tissue in the breast can form a cancer, but usually it comes from either the ducts or the glands. Cancers may be invasive or non-invasive. Over the course of a lifetime, one in eight women will be diagnosed with breast cancer.

Calcium-D-Glucarate - The calcium salt of D-glucaric acid, a natural substance found in many fruits and vegetables. One of the key ways in which the body eliminates toxic chemicals, as well as hormones such as estrogen, is by attaching glucuronic acid to them in the liver and then excreting this complex in the bile.

Candida – A yeast-like fungi commonly found in nature. Species can be isolated from the skin, vaginal, and pharyngeal tissues, as well as the gastrointestinal tract.

Carcinogenic – Any cancer-producing substance or organism.

Castration – Removal of the ovaries or testicles, or gonadal atrophy produced by prolonged treatment with sex hormones.

Catalyze – To act as a catalyst: a substance that accelerates a chemical reaction but is not consumed or changed permanently.

Cell – The smallest unit of living structure capable of independent existence.

Cell Proliferation - An increase in the number of cells as a result of cell growth and cell division.

Cervix – The lower part of the uterus extending from the isthmus of the uterus into the vagina.

Cessation – To stop action, to discontinue.

Cholesterol – The most abundant steroid in animal tissues, this substance is an essential component of cell membranes and nerve fiber insulation. Cholesterol is important for the metabolism and transport of fatty acids and in the production of hormones and Vitamin D. Cholesterol is manufactured by the liver, and is also present in certain foods (e.g., eggs, shellfish, animal fat). There are 2 types of cholesterol in the blood, high-density (HDL) and low-density (LDL) lipoproteins. Very low cholesterol levels may indicate malnutrition.

Chronic – A health-related state lasting a long time. A chronic condition is one that lasts 3 months or longer.

Coagulation – Clotting; the process of changing from a liquid to a solid or semisolid mass (gel).

Colorectal Cancer – Colon and rectal cancer have many features in common and are often referred to together as colorectal cancer. Colon and rectal cancers begin in the digestive system, also called the GI (gastrointestinal) system. This is where food is changed to create energy and rid the body of waste matter. Over 95% of colon and rectal cancers are adenocarcinomas. These are cancers of the cells that line the inside of the colon and rectum.

Conjugated – Joined or paired. The joining together of two compounds.

Coronary Heart Disease - Heart disease is caused by narrowing of the coronary arteries that feed the heart. If not enough oxygen-carrying blood reaches the heart, you may experience chest pain called angina. If the blood supply to a portion of the heart is completely cut off by total blockage of a coronary artery, the result is a heart attack. This is usually due to a sudden closure from a blood clot forming on top of a previous narrowing.

Cortisol - Cortisol is the most potent glucocorticoid produced by the human adrenal. It is synthesized from cholesterol and its production is stimulated by pituitary adrenocorticotropic hormone (ACTH). Cortisol affects immune function, glucose counter regulation, vascular tone, and bone metabolism.

Cruciferous - Cruciferous is the scientific name for a group of plants whose four petal flowers resemble a cross. These vegetables are a part of the cabbage family and include arugula, bok choy, broccoli, broccoli sprouts, Brussels sprouts, cabbage, cauliflower, Swiss chard, collards, kale, kohlrabi, mustard greens, radishes, rutabaga, turnips, turnip greens, and watercress.

Data and Safety Monitoring Board (DSMB) – Sometimes called an Independent Data Safety Monitoring Board. It has the responsibility of terminating clinical trial subjects, clinical trial methods, or the trial itself in order to protect the subjects. It analyzes clinical trial results at frequent intervals to determine if undue risks to subject safety are developing. The DSMB protects patients, and ensures that the protocol remains adequate to answer the questions originally posed by the study. A DSMB is not mandated by federal regulations, and is not present in every clinical trial. A DSMB is more likely to be present where an unusually high degree of clinical knowledge may be necessary to evaluate possible dangers.

Dehydroepiandrosterone (DHEA) – A hormone with both androgenic and estrogenic effects, and one of the precursors of testosterone. It is primarily secreted by the adrenal glands.

Dementia – The progressive loss of cognitive and intelligence functions without impairment of perception or consciousness. Characterized by disorientation as well as impaired memory, judgement, and intellect.

Depression – A temporary mental state or chronic mental disorder characterized by feelings of sadness, loneliness, despair, low self-esteem, and self-reproach.

Diindolymethane (D.I.M.) - An indole plant nutrient found in cruciferous vegetables including broccoli, cabbage, brussels sprouts and cauliflower. Diindolylmethane supports the activity of specific enzymes that improve estrogen metabolism. Scientific research shows diindolylmethane increases the level of "good" estrogens (2-hydroxyestrogcn) while reducing the level of "bad" estrogens (16-hydroxyestrogen).

Dual Energy X-Ray Absorptionmetry Scan (DEXA) - The most sensitive instrument used to measure bone mass. The machine passes an X-ray beam through an area of the bone using ultrasound sound waves instead of X-rays. Radiation or sound waves are absorbed by the bone, with the result being that the denser the bone, the more it absorbs. The DEXA scan is very accurate and can measure some changes in bone density. This is the preferred test for osteoporosis screening.

Dysfunction – Abnormal function.

Efficacy – The extent to which a specific intervention, procedure, regimen, or service produces a beneficial result.

Endocrine System – The anatomical system made up of ductless glands: adrenal glands, ovaries, parathyroid glands, pancreas, pineal gland, pituitary gland, testes, thyroid gland, thymus.

Endometrial Cancer - Endometrial cancer is a cancer that develops from the endometrium, the inner lining of the uterus (womb).

Endometriosis - When the inner lining of the uterus (womb) becomes inflamed during the menstrual cycle.

Enzyme – A protein that acts as a catalyst to induce chemical changes in other substances, remaining unchanged in the process.

Epinephrine – Commonly known as adrenalin. Epinephrine is a catecholamine secreted by the adrenal glands in response to low blood glucose, exercise, and stress. Epinephrine causes a breakdown of glycogen to glucose in the liver, encourages the release of fatty acids from adipose tissue (fat cells), causes widening of the small arteries within muscle, and increases cardiac output. Heightened secretion caused perhaps by fear or anger will result in increased heart rate and the hydrolysis of glycogen to glucose; this reaction is often called the "fight or flight" response.

Equilibrium – Being evenly balanced. A state of repose between two or more antagonistic forces that exactly counteract each other.

Equiline – An estrogenic steroid occurring in the urine of pregnant mares (horses).

Equinal - An estrogenic steroid occurring in the urine of pregnant mares (horses).

Estradiol – The most potent naturally occurring estrogen in mammals. Formed by the ovaries and the placenta.

Estriol – An estrogenic metabolite of estradiol.

Estrogen – Generic term for any substance (natural or synthetic) that exerts biological effects characteristic of estrogenic hormones.

Estrogen/Medroxyprogesterone Tablets - Prempro, Premphase.

Estrogen Deficient - The body lacks normal estrogen levels.

Estrogen Dominance – The body has too much estrogen in relation to progesterone.

Estrogenic – Causing estrus in animals. Having an action similar to that of an estrogen.

Estrone – A metabolite of estradiol.

Evidenced – Supported by evidence. That which is manifested.

Exogenous – Originating or produced outside of the organism.

Fibrocystic Disease - Benign changes in the breast, with no suggestion of any cancer in the biopsies. Extra fibrous tissue or hardening of the breast tissue that feels lumpy. The risk of benign breast disease turning into cancer is very limited.

Fibroid Tumor - A non-cancerous growth, consisting of fibrous and muscular tissue, especially occurring in the uterus. It can occur inside the cavity, inside the wall and on the outer surface.

Fibromyalgia – Pain in the muscles and in the fibrous connective tissues but uncertain cause. Fibromyalgia is a syndrome characterized by musculoskeletal pain and tenderness at specified sites, fatigue, unrefreshing sleep, and multiple systemic symptoms.

Follicle – A spherical-shaped mass of cells that usually contains a cavity.

Follicle-Stimulating Hormone (FSH) - Synthesized in the pituitary gland. In sexually mature females, FSH (assisted by Luteinizing Hormone) acts on the follicle to stimulate it to release estrogens.

Genitalia – The organs used for reproduction.

Gestation – Pregnancy. The period of fetal development in the uterus from conception to birth.

Gonadotropin - A hormone that can stimulate the testicles to produce sperm or the ovaries to produce an egg.

Gynecologist - A physician who specializes in the diseases and the routine physical care of the reproductive system of women. Not the same as a reproductive endocrinologist, who is a gynecologist with additional specialization in infertility and assisted reproductive technology.

Gynecology – The medical specialty concerned with the diseases of the female genital tract, as well as endocrinology and reproductive physiology of the female.

Heart Palpitations - Palpitations are an uncomfortable awareness of your heartbeat. Feeling as if one's heart is beating harder or faster than usual or skipping a beat or two, a perception of irregularity of the pulse, uneasiness or a flip-flopping in the chest. Quite often palpitations are associated with lightheadedness or even loss of consciousness.

Hepatic – Relating to the liver.

Holistic Medicine - A system of health care leading towards optimal attainment of the physical, mental, emotional, social, and spiritual aspects of health. It emphasizes the need to look at the whole person, including analysis of physical, nutritional, environmental, emotional, social, spiritual, and lifestyle values.

Hormone – A chemical substance formed in one organ or part of the body and carried in the blood to another organ or part. Most hormones are formed in the ductless glands.

Hormone Replacement Therapy (HRT) – A treatment for women having reached or passed menopause. HRT involves taking small doses of one or two hormones, estrogen and progesterone.

Human-Identical – Means "exactly the same," "identical" to the molecule produced by the human body.

Hypo-Estrogenic Amenorrhea - An absence of menstruation due to low estrogen levels caused by low levels of pituitary hormones.

Hysterectomy – Usually involves the complete removal of the uterus, unless otherwise specified. Types of hysterectomies: Partial Hysterectomy, Supra-Cervical Hysterectomy, Oophorectomy, Bi-Lateral Salpingo-Oophorectomy, Complete Hysterectomy, Total Abdominal Hysterectomy with Bi-Lateral Salpingo-Oophorectomy.

Immune Response - The body's ability to defend against foreign substances that invade it or are introduced into it.

Incontinence – Inability to prevent the discharge of urine and/or feces. There may be an actual loss of urine involved or merely the threatened loss (or urge).

Insomnia – One's inability to sleep with regularity.

Lethargy – Reduced alertness and awareness.

Libido – Conscious or unconscious sexual desire.

Luteinizing Hormone (LH) - Synthesized in the pituitary gland. In sexually mature females, LH stimulates the follicle to secrete estrogen in the first half of the menstrual cycle. Also stimulates the follicle to secrete progesterone during the latter half of the menstrual cycle.

Mammogram – Radiological examination of the female breast to screen for cancer.

Medroxyprogesterone Acetate – A synthetic derivative of progesterone. Brand name is Provera.

Menopause – Permanent cessation of the menstrual cycle.

Menstrual Cycle – Refers to the monthly cyclical changes in endocrine levels and their effects on follicular development and the uterine endometrial cycle. This cycle starts at puberty and ceases at menopause.

Mercurial – Having the characteristic of rapidly changing moods.

Metabolic Pathways – The chemical and biochemical processes of metabolism.

Metabolism – The chemical and physical changes occurring in living tissue to acquire and utilize energy.

Metabolite – Any product of metabolism.

Metamorphosis – A change in form, structure, or function. The transition from one developing stage to another. A transformation.

Micronutrient Metal – Essential metals found in foods that are required in small amounts by the body.

Migraine – Also known as a vascular headache. Is caused by dilation or swelling of blood vessels inside and outside the scalp in people who have very sensitive blood vessels. Dialation allows more blood to pump through the vessels, causing a throbbing. Migraines can take several different forms, but the pain is usually extreme and preceded by altered vision followed by nausea and vomiting.

Natural Menopause - When a woman has not had a menstrual period for a full year and menstruation has permanently ended without any kind of medical intervention, natural menopause has been reached. Menopause is a change that is a natural and normal occurrence.

Neurotransmitter – A chemical messenger used by an organism to communicate among neurons and between neurons and other types of cells.

Norethindrone Acetate - Second Generation Progestin, this synthetic progestational hormone (trade name Norlutin) is used in oral contraceptives to treat endometriosis and may also be used to treat menstrual disorders.

Obstetrician – A physician specializing in the medical care of women during pregnancy and childbirth.

Organic Chemistry - The study of carbon-containing compounds and their properties.

Osteoporosis – A reduction in the quantity of bone or atrophy of skeletal tissue. Usually an age-related disorder characterized by decreased bone mass.

Ovaries – The pair of female reproductive glands containing the ova (egg) or germ cells.

Ovulation – Release of an ovum from the ovarian follicle.

PAP Smear - A procedure in which a specimen of cells is taken from the uterine cervix and examined for abnormal cell growth.

Perimenopause – Means around menopause. This is a transition phase coming before menopause and may last from two to eight years. Women in this lifecycle are typically late forties to early fifties.

Pharmacology – The scientific study of drugs, their sources, appearance, chemistry, actions, and uses.

Pharmacotherapy – The treatment of disease by the use of drugs.

Pituitary Gland – Considered the master endocrine gland. It is about the size of a pea and located beneath the hypothalamus in a bony cavity at the base of the skull. Its secretes many hormones, including thyroid-stimulating hormone, adrenocorticotropic hormone (ACTH), gonadotropins, growth hormone, prolactin, lipotropin, melanocyte-stimulating hormone, antidiuretic hormone (ADH), oxytocin, LH, and FSH.

Premarin – A conjugated estrogen product extracted from pregnant mare's urine. Manufactured by Wyeth-Ayerst Pharmaceuticals.

Postmenopausal – Relating to the period of time following menopause.

Premenopausal – Relating to the period of time preceding menopause.

Premenstrual Syndrome (PMS) - The group of symptoms related to the menstrual cycle and occurring one or two weeks before menses.

Prempro – A combination of conjugated horse estrogen and progestin (synthetic progesterone) together. Manufactured by Wyeth-Ayerst Pharmaceuticals.

Progesterone – An antiestrogenic steroid, this hormone is secreted by the ovaries and the adrenal glands and is considered as important in a woman's reproductive system as estrogen.

Progesterone Balance - A normal level of progesterone in relation to estrogen.

Progesterone/Estradiol Ratio (Pg/E2) - The proper balance between these two hormones.

Provera – A synthetic progestin: medroxyprogesterone.

Steroids – The family of chemical substances containing the tetracyclic cyclopenta[a]phenanthrene skeleton. Comprised of many hormones, body constituents, and drugs.

Stroke – Occurs when blood vessels carrying oxygen and nutrients to the brain are either blocked by a clot or burst, thus impairing cerebral circulation for more than 24 hours.

Sublingual - Under the tongue.

Surgical Menopause – The resulting hormonal condition caused by the surgical removal of both ovaries or one ovary and the uterus.

Synthetic – Made by synthesis. Not natural.

T-Score - Developed because of variation in BMD measurement technology among different manufacturers. The number of standard deviations the bone mineral density measurement is above or below the Young-Normal Mean mineral density.

Testosterone – Believed to be the most potent naturally occuring androgen. A vital sex hormone that plays an important role in puberty. Testosterone isn't exclusively a male hormone. Women produce small amounts of it in their bodies as well.

Therapeutic –Relating to the treatment, remediating, or curing of a disorder or disease.

Triest - Triple estrogen: Triest is the name of the bio-identical hormone that is frequently given to women with acute menopausal symptoms. Contains estriol, estradiol, and estrone.

Triglycerides - The main type of fat transported by your body.

Uterus – The uterus is a pear-shaped organ located between the bladder and lower intestine. It consists of two parts: the corpus (body) and the cervix (neck). When a woman is not pregnant, the body of the uterus is about the size of a fist.

Vagina – The genital canal in the female, extending from the uterus the vulva.

Vasomotor – Causing dilation or constriction of the blood vessels.

Z-Score - Developed because of variation in BMD measurement technology among different manufacturers. The number of standard deviations in the measurement is above or below the Age-Matched Mean bone mineral density.

References

Chapter 1

Hasson, H. (1993). Cervical removal at hysterectomy for benign disease. *Journal of Reproductive Medicine, 58*, (10) 781-789.

Lee, John R. M.D. (1996). *What Your Doctor May Not Tell You About Menopause.* New York. Warner Books, 14.

Massoudi, M.S., et. Al. (1995). Prevalence of thyroid antibodies among healthy middle age women. Findings from the study in healthy women. *Annals of Epidemiology*, 5 (3), 229-233.

Northrup, Christiane, M.D. (2001). *The Wisdom of Menopause.* New York. Bantam Books, 111.

Wright, J.V., M.D., and Morgenthaler, J. (1997). *Natural Hormone Replacement*; CA, Smart Publications, 51.

Chapter 2

Bhavnai, B. (1998). Pharmacokinetics and pharmacodynamics of conjugated equine estrogens: Chemistry and metabolism. *Proceedings of the Society for Biological Medicine, 217* (1), 6-16.

Cole, W., et al. (1995, June 26). The estrogen dilemma. *Time*, 46-53 (cover story).

Consumer Advisory. National Center for Complementary Medicine. (2002). Alternative Therapies for Managing Menopausal Symptoms. http://wwwnccam.nih.gov

Crews JK, Khalil RA. (1999). Antagonistic effects of 17 -estradiol, progesterone, and testosterone on Ca ++ entry mechanisms of coronary vasoconstriction. *Arteriosclerosis, Thrombosis, and Vascular Biology 19*:1034-1040.

Daly, E., et al. (1996). Risk of venus thromboembolism in users of hormone replacement therapy. *Lancet, 348*, 977-980.

Follingingstad, A. (1978). Estriol, the forgotton hormone. *The Journal of the American Medical Association, 239 (1),* 29-39.

Fugh-Berman, A. MD., and Cynthia Pearson, BS. (2002) The Overselling of Hormone Replacement Therapy. *Pharmacotherapy 22* (9): 1205-1208.

Gillson, G. R., and Zava, D. T. (2003). 2003 Perspective on Hormone Replacement for Women: Picking up the pieces after the Women's Health Initiative Trial. *International Journal of Pharmaceutical Compounding, 7* (4), 250.

Grodstein, F., et al. (1996). Prospective study of exogenous hormones and risk of pulmonary embolism in women. *Lancet, 348,* 983-986.

Grodstein, F., Newcomb, P. A., and Stampfer, M. J. (1999). Postmenopausal hormone therapy and the risk of colorectal cancer. A review and meta-analysis. *The American Journal of Medicine, 106* (5), 574-582.

Hully, S., et al. (1998). Randomized trial of estrogen plus progestin for secondary prevention of coronary heart disease in post menopausal women. *The Journal of the American Medical Association, 280,* 605-618.

Jick, H., et al. (1996). Risk of hospital admissions for idiopathic venous thromboembolism among users of postmenopausal estrogen. *Lancet, 348,* 981-986.

Lemon, H. (1975). Estriol prevention of mammary carcinoma induced by 7,12-dimethylbenzathracene and procarbazine. *Cancer Research, 35,* 1341-1353.

Lemon, H. (1973). Orstriol and prevention of breast cancer. *Lancet, 1,* (802), 546-547.

Lemon, H. (1980). Pathophysiologic considerations in the treatment of menopausal patients with oestrogens: The role of oestriol in the prevention of mammary cancer.

Acta Endocrinologica, 233, suppl., 17-27.

Lemon, H., Wotiz, H., Parsons., et al. (1966). Reduced estriol excretion in patients with breast cancer prior to endocrine therapy. *The Journal of the American Medical Association*, 196, 1128-136.

Mauldin, Robert K. (1999). New HRT approved. *Modern Medicine, 67* (7), 55, 2p.

Mayo Foundation for Medical Education and Research (2003). Hormone replacement therapy: Who should take it and what are the alternatives? Online. Internet. http://www.Mayoclinic.com.

Mosca, L. (2000). The role of hormone replacement therapy in the prevention of postmenopausal heart disease. *Archives of Internal Medicine, 160*, 2263-2272.

North Americal Menopause Society (2003). FDA Approves New Labels for Estrogen and Estrogin with Progestin Therapies for Postmenopausal Women. Online.Internet. http//: www.menopause.org

Reuters. More Bad News for Hormone Drugs in U.S. Study. (2003). Conlon, Michael. Http://www.1800lawinfo.com

Sarrel, P. (1999). The differential effects of oestrogens and progestins on vascular tone. *Human Reproduction Update, 5* (3), 205-209.

Shen, L., Qiu, S., Chen, Y., Ahang, F., van Breemen, R. B., Nikoliv, D., & Bolton, J. L. (1998). Alkylation of 2-deoxynucleosides and DNA by Prearin metabolite 4-hydroxyequilenin semiquinone radical. *Chemical Research in Toxicology, 11*, 94-101.

Sullivan, J. M., et al. (1995). Progestin enhances vasoconstrictor responses in postmenopausal women receiving estrogen replacement therapy. *Menopause, 4*, 193-197.

The Postmenopausal Estrogen/Progestin Intervention (PEPI) trial (1995). Effects of estrogen or estrogen/progestin regimens on heart disease risk factors in postmenopausal women. *The Journal of the American Medical Association, 273,* 199-206.

Williame, J. K., et al. (1994). Effects of hormone replacement therapy on reactivity of atherosclerotic coronary arteries in cynomologous monkeys, *Journal of the American College of Cardiology, 24,* 1757-1761.

Women's Health Initiative (2004). Effects of Conjugated Equine Estrogen in Postmenopausal Women with Hysterectomy. *The Journal of the American Medical Association, 291*:1701-1712.

Yaffe, K., Lui, L.Y., Grady, D., Cauley, J., Kramer, J., & Cummings, S. R. (2000). Cognitive decline in women in relation to non-protein-bound estradiol concentractions. *Lancet, 356* (9231), 708-712.

Zhang, F., et al. (1999). The major metabolite of equilin, 4-hydroxyequilin, autoxidies to an o-quinone which isomerizes to the potent cytotoxin 4-hydroxyequinone-o-quinone. *Chemical Research in Toxicology, 12,* 204-213.

Chapter 3

Gavin, N., Thorp, J., and Oshfeldt, R. (2001). Determinants of hormone replacement therapy duration among postmenopausal women with intact uteri. *Menopause, 8,* 377-383.

Gillson, G. R., and Zava, D. T. (2003). 2003 Perspective on Hormone Replacement for Women: Picking up the pieces after the Women's Health Initiative Trial. *International Journal of Pharmaceutical Compounding, 7* (4), 250.

Mosby. (1998). Human Pharmocology, Third Edition. Mosby-Year Book, Inc., St. Louis, Missouri.

National Institutes of Health News Release. (July 9, 2002). NLHBI Stops Trial of Estrogen Plus Progestin Due to Increased Breast Cancer Risk, Lack of Overall Benefit.

The Writing Group for the Women's Health Initiative. (2002). Risks and benefits of estrogen plus progestin in healthy post-menopausal women. *The Journal of the American Medical Association, 288*:321-333.

Jonathan V. Wright, M.D. and John Morgenthaler. (1997). *Natural Hormone Replacement*, Smart Publications, CA 23.

Wright JV. (1999). Comparative measurements of serum estriol, estradiol, and E1 in non-pregnant, premenopausal women; A preliminary investigation. *Alternative Medicine Review ;4*, 266-270.

Schechter D. (1999). Estrogen, progesterone, and mood. *Journal of Gender-Specific Medicine (2)*, 29-36.

Chapter 4

Graham JD, and Clarke CL. (1997). Physiological action of pro-gesterone in target tissues. *Endocrine Reviews 18 (4)*, 502-519.

Wright JV. (1999). Comparative measurements of serum estriol, estradiol, and E1 in non-pregnant, premenopausal women; A preliminary investigation. *Alternative Medicine Review, (4)* , 266-270.

Schechter D. (1999). Estrogen, progesterone, and mood. *Journal of Gender-Specific Medicine ;2*, 29-36.

Chapter 5

Aardal E, Holm AC. (1995). Cortisol in saliva-reference ranges and relation to cortisol in serum. *European Journal of Clinical Chemistry and Clinical Biochemistry, 33*, 927-932.

Aardal-Eriksson E, Karlberg BE, Holm AC. (1998). Salivary cortisol- and alternative to serum cortisol determinations in dynamic function tests. *Clinical Chemistry and Laboratory Medicine, 36*, 215-222.

Allolio B, Hoffmann J, Linton EA, Winkelmann W, Kusche M, Schulte HM. (1990). Diurnal salivary cortisol patterns during pregnancy and after delivery: relationship to plasma corticotrophin-releasing hormone. *Clinical Endocrinology, 33*, 279-289.

Barrou Z, Guiban D, Maroufi A, Fournier C, Dugue MA, Luton JP, Thomopoulos P. (1996). Overnight dexamethasone suppression test: comparison of plasma and salivary cortisol measurement for the screening of Cushing's syndrome. *European Journal of Endocrinology, 134*,93-96.

Bolaji II, Tallon DF, O'Dwyer E, Fottrell PF. (1993). Assessment of bioavailability of oral micronized progesterone using a salivary progesterone enzymeimmunoassay. *Gynecological Endocrinology, 7*, 101-110.

Booth A, Johnson D, Granger D, Crouter A, McHale S. Testosterone and child and adolescent adjustment: the moderating role of parent-child relationships. October 2000. Unpublished manuscript.

Campbell BC, Ellison PT. (1992). Menstrual variation in salivary testosterone among regularly cycling women. *Hormone Research, 37*, 132-136.

Castro M, Elias PC, Quidute AR, Halah FP, Moreira AC. (1999). Out-patient screening for Cushing's Syndrome: the sensitivity of the combination of circadian rhythm and overnight dexamethasone suppression salivary cortisol tests. *The Journal of Clinical Endocrinology & Metabolism, 84*, 878-882.

Choe JK, Khan-Dawood FS, Dawood MY. (1983). Progesterone and estradiol in the saliva and plasma during the menstrual cycle. *American Journal of Obstetrics and Gynecology, 147*, 557-562.

Dabbs JM. (1991). Salivary testosterone measurements: collecting, storing and mailing saliva samples. *Physiology and Behavior, 49*, 815-817.

Dabbs JM. (1990). Salivary testosterone measurements: reliability across hours, days and weeks. *Physiology and Behavior, 49,* 48: 83-86.

Dabbs JM, Campbell BC, Gladue BA, Midgley AR, Navarro MA, Read GF, Susman EJ, Swinkels LM, Worthman CM. (1995). Reliability of salivary testosterone measurements: a multicenter evaluation. *Clinical Chemistry* , 41, 1581-1584.

Delfs TM, Klein S, Fottrell P, Naether OG, Leidenberger FA, Zimmermann RC. (1994). 24-Hour profiles of salivary progesterone. *Fertility and Sterility, 62*, 960-966.

Filaire E, Duche P, Lac G, Robert A. (1996). Saliva cortisol, physical exercise and training: influences of swimming and handball on cortisol concentrations in women. *European Journal of Applied Physiology, 74*, 274-278.

Filaire E, Lac G. (2000). Dehydroepiandrosterone (DHEA) rather than testosterone shows saliva androgen responses to exercise in elite female handball players. *International Journal of Sports Medicine, 21*, 17-20.

Finn MM, Gosling JP, Tallon DF, Baynes S, Meehan FP, Fottrell PF. (1992). The frequency of salivary progesterone sampling and the diagnosis of luteal phase insufficiency. *Gynecological Endocrinology, 6*, 127-134.

Heine RP, McGregor JA, Dullien VK. (1999). Accuracy of salivary estriol testing compared to traditional risk factor assessment in predicting preterm birth. *American Journal of Obstetrics and Gynecology*, 180, S214-218.

Khan-Dawood FS, Choe JK, Dawood MY. (1984). Salivary and plasma bound and "free" testosterone in men and women. *American Journal of Obstetrics and Gynecology, 148*, 441-445.

Kudielka BM, Schmidt-Reinwald AK, Hellhammer DH, Kirschbaum C. (1999). Psychological and endocrine responses to psychosocial stress and dexamethasone/corticotropin-releasing hormone in healthy postmenopausal women and young controls: the impact of age and a two-week estradiol treatment. *Neuroendocrinology, 70*, 422-430.

Lac G, Lac N, Robert A. (1993). Steroid assays in saliva: a method to detect plasmatic contaminations. *Archives of International Physiology, Biochemistry, and Biophysics, 101*, 257-262.

Lipson SF, Ellison PT. (1992). Normative study of age variation in salivary progesterone profiles. *Journal of Biosocial Science*, 24, 233-244.

Lipson SF, Ellison PT. Development of protocols for the application of salivary steroid analyses to field conditions. *American Journal of Human Biology, 1*, 249-255.

Lo MS, Ng ML, Azmy BS, Khalid BA. (1992). Clinical applications of salivary cortisol measurements. *Singapore Medical Journal, 33*, 170.

Lu Y, Bentley GR, Gann PH, Hodges KR, Chatterton RT. (1999). Salivary estradiol and progesterone levels in conception and nonconception cycles in women: evaluation of a new assay for salivary estradiol. *Fertility and Sterility, 71*, 863-868.

Lu YC, Chatterton RT, Vogelsong KM, May LK. (1997). Direct radioimmunoassay of progesterone in saliva. *Journal of Immunoassay, 18*, 149-163.

Navarro MA, Nolla JM, Machuca MI, Gonzalez A, Mateo L, Bonnin RM, Roig-Escofet D. (1998). Salivary testosterone in postmenopausal women with rheumatoid arthritis. *The Journal of Rheumatology, 25*, 1059-1062.

O'Rourke MT, Ellison PT. (1993). Salivary estradiol levels decrease with age in healthy, regularly-cycling women. *Endocrinology, 1*, 487-494.

Petsos P, Ratcliffe WA, Heath DF, Anderson DC. (1986). Comparison of blood spot, salivary and serum progesterone assays in the normal menstrual cycle. *Clinical Endocrinology, 24*, 31-38.

Quissell D. (1993). Steroid hormone analysis in human saliva. *Annals of the New York Academy of Sciences*, 694, 143-145.

Raff H, Raff JL, Findling JW. (1998). Late-night salivary cortisol as a screening test for Cushing's Syndrome. *Journal of Clinical Endocrinology & Metabolism*, 83, 2681-2686.

Read GF. (1993). Status report on measurement of salivary estrogens and androgens. *Annals of the New York Academy of Sciences,* September 20; 694: 146-160.

Read GF, Wilson DW, Campbell FC, Holliday HW, Blamey RW, Griffiths K. (1983). Salivary cortisol and dehydroepiandrosterone sulphate levels in postmenopausal women with primary breast cancer. *European Journal of Cancer and Clinical Oncology, 19*, 477-483.

Scheer FA, Buijs RM. (1999). Light affects morning salivary cortisol in humans. *Journal of Clinical Endocrinology, 84*, 3395-3398.

Steptoe A, Cropley M, Griffith J, Kirschbaum C. (2000). Job strain and anger expression predict early morning elevation in salivary cortisol. *Psychosomatic Medicine, 62*, 286-292.

Sumiala S, Tuominen J, Huhtaniemi I, Maenpaa J. (1996). Salivary progesterone concentrations after tubal sterilization. *Obstetrics & Gynecology, 88*, 792-796.

Swinkels LM, Ross HA, Smals AG, Benraad TJ. (1990). Concentrations of total and free dehydroepiandrosterone in plasma and dehydroepiandrosterone in saliva of normal and hirsute women under basal conditions and during administration of dexamethasone/synthetic corticotropin. *Clinical Chemistry, 16*, 2042-2046.

Tschop M, Behre HM, Nieschlag E, Dressendorfer RA, Strasburger CJ. (1998). A time-resolved fluorescence immunoassay for the measurement of testosterone in saliva: monitoring of testosterone replacement therapy with testosterone buciclate. *Clinical Chemistry Laboratory Medicine, 36*, 223-230.

Vail, Jane. (2003). "Natural" or "Bioidentical" Hormone Replacement: What Makes the Difference? An Interview with Christopher B. Cutter, MD. International Journal of Pharmaceutical Compounding, 7 (1).

Vining RF, McGinley RA, Symons RG. (1983). Hormones in saliva: mode of entry and consequent implications for clinical interpretation. *Clinical Chemistry, 29*, 1752-1756.

Vining RF, McGinley RA. (1987). The measurement of hormones in saliva: possibilities and pitfalls. *Journal of Steroid Biochemistry, 27* (1-3), 81-94.

Vittek J, L'Hommedieu D, Gordon G, Rappaport S, Southren L. (1985). Direct radioimmunoassay (RIA) of salivary testosterone: correlation with free and total serum testosterone. *Life Sciences* *37*, 711-716.

Voss HF. (1999). Saliva as a fluid for measurement of estradiol levels. *American Journal of Obstetrics and Gynecology, 180*, S226-231.

Wang DY, Fantl VE, Habibollahi F, Clark GM, Fentiman IS, Hayward JL, Bulbrook RD. (1986). Salivary oestradiol and progesterone levels in premenopausal women with breast cancer. *European Journal of Cancer and Clinical Oncology, Apr, 22* (4), 427-33.

Wang DY, Knyba RE. (1985). Salivary progesterone: relation to total and non-protein-bound blood levels. *Journal of Steroid Biochemistry, 23*, 975-979.

Worthman CM, Stallings JF, Hofman LF. (1990). Sensitive salivary estradiol assay for monitoring ovarian function. *Clinical Chemistry, 36*, 1769-1773.

Wren B, McFarland K, Edwards L, O'Shea P, Sufi S et al. (2000). Effect of sequential transdermal progesterone cream on endometrium, bleeding pattern, and plasma progesterone and salivary progesterone levels in postmenopausal women. *Climacteric 3*, 155-160.

Wright Jonathan V. M.D., Margenthaler J. (1997). *How To Obtain Natural Hormones. Natural Hormone Replacement*, Smart Publications, 115-117.

Chapter 6

Bachman, D.L. (1992). Sleep Disorders with Aging: Evaluation and Treatment. *Geriatrics 47, 9*, 53-61.

Bachmann G.A., et al. (1999). Female Sexuality During the Menopause. *OBG Management suppl. 11(5)*.

Bales L. (1998). Treatment of the Perimenopausal Female. *Primary Care Update Ob/Gyns 5, 2*,90-94.

Cauley J.A., Lucas F.L., Kuller L.H., et al. (1996). Bone Mineral Density and Risk of Breast Cancer in Older Women: The Study of Osteoporotic Fractures. *The Journal of the American Medical Association 276*, 1404.

Clardson T.B. (2000). The Effects of Hormone Replacement Therapy on Key Factors for Cardiovascular Disease. *Hormone Replacement Therapy Cardiovascular Health.* Fairlawn, NJ: MPE Commuications.

Dennerstein L., et al. (1979). Sexuality, hormones and the menopause transition. *Maturitas 26*, 83-93.

DeSouzaM.J., Prestwood K.M., Luciano A.A., Miller B.E., Nulsen J.C. (1996). A Comparison of the Effect of Synthetic and Micronized Hormone Replacement Therapy on Bone Mineral Density and Biochemical Markers of Bone Metabolism. *Journal of the North American Menopausal Society 3*, 140.

Gilson G.R. M.D., Ph.D., Zava D.T.,PhD. (2003). A Perspective on HRT for Women: Picking Up The Pieces After the Women's Health Initiative Trial, Part 2. *International Journal of Pharmaceutical Compounding, 7(5)*, 330-338.

Heart Disease Is The Number 1 Killer of Women in the United States. (1998). *Heart Strong Women.* The American College of Obstetricians and Gynecologists.

Koefoed P., Brahm J. (1994). The permeability of the human red cell membrane to steroid sex hormones. *Biochimica et Biophysics Acta, 1195*, 55-62.

Lindsay R. (1993). Prevention and Treatment of Osteoporosis. *Lancet 341*, 801.

Molinari C, Battaglia A, Grossini E et al. (2001). Effect of progesterone on peripheral blood flow in prepubertal female anesthetized pigs. *Journal of Vascular Research, 38,*569-577.

Newton K.M., LaCroix A.Z. (1999). Hormone Replacement Therapy and Tertiary Prevention of Coronary Heart Disease. *Menopausal Medicine 7, (2),*5-8.

NIH Concensus Development Panel. (2001). Osteoporosis Prevention, Diagnosis, and Therapy. *The Journal of the American Medical Association 285*, 785

Randolph C.W. Jr. M.D., (1999). *Natural Hormone Balance.* Jacksonville, FL. Women's Medicine, Inc.

Rosano G.M., Webb C.M., Chierchia S et al. (2000). Natural progesterone, but not medroxyprogesterone acetate, enhances the beneficial effect of estrogen on exercise-induced myocardial ischemia in postmenopausal women. *Journal of the American College of Cardiology, 36*, 2154-2159.

Schwartz E., M.D. (2002). *The Hormone Solution.* New York: Warner Books.

Sherwin B.B. (1997). Estrogen Effects of Cognition on Menopausal Women. *Neurology 48 suppl.,* S21-S26.

Sotelo M., Johnson S.R. (1997). The Effects of Hormone Replacement Therapy on Coronary Heart Disease. *Endocrinology and Metabolism Clinics of North America 26 (2)*, 313-327.

Speroff L. (2001). Hormone Replacement Therapy: Clarifying the Picture. *Hospital Practice.* http://www.hosppract.com/issues/2001/05/dmmspe.htm

Speroff L. (1997). Postmenopausal Hormone Therapy and Cardiovascular System. Oregon Health Services University School of Medicine. *Contemporary Ob/Gyn, 426.*

Speroff L. (1998). The Heart and Estrogen/Progestin Replacement Study (HERS). *Maturitas,* Vol 31, Issue 3, pg 9.

Spiegel K, Leproult R, Van Cauter E. (1999). Impact of Sleep Debt in Metabolic and Endocrine Function. *Lancet 354,*1435-1439.

Taskinen M.R., et al. (1996). Hormone Replacement Therapy Lowers Plasma Lp(a) Concentrations, Comparison Cyclic Transdermal and Continuous Estrogen Progestin Regimens. *Arteriosclerosis, Thrombosis, and Vascular Biology, 16,* 1215-1221.

Washburn S.A. (1997). Estradiol and Progesterone Effects on the Central Nervous System. *Menopausal Medicine 5(4),*5-8.

Waddell B.J., Leary P.C.O. (2001). Distribution and metabolism of topically applied progesterone in a rat model. *Journal of Steroid Biochemistry and Molecular Biology, 80,* 449-455.

Whitcroft S.I., Crook D, Marsh M.S., et al. (1994). Long Term Effects of Oral and Transdermal Hormone Replacement Therapies on Serum Lipid and Lipoprotein Concentrations. *Obstetrics and Gynecology, 84,* 222.

Williams J.K., Honore E.K., Washburn SA et al. (1994). Effects of hormone replacement therapy on reactivity of artherosclerotic coronary arteries in cynomolgus monkeys. *Journal of the American College of Cardiology, 224,* 1757-1761

Zhang Y., et al. (1998). Bone Mass and the Risk of Cancer Among Postmenopausal Women. *New England Journal of Medicine, 336,* 611-617.

Chapter 7

Cummings S.R., Black D.M., Rubin S.M. (1989). Lifetime risk of hip. Colles: or vertebral fracture and coronary heart disease among white postmenopausal women. *Archives of Internal Medicine, 149,* 2445-2448.

Faulkner K.G., von Stecten E., Miller P. (1999). Discordance in patient classification using T-scores. *Journal of Clinical Densitometry, 2,* 343-350.

Bonnick S.L., Johnson C.C. Jr., Kleerekoper M., et al. (2001). Importance of precision in bone density measurements. *Journal of Clinical Densitometry,* 105-110.

Facts on Osteoporosis and Related Bone Diseases. (2002). National Resource Center, National Institutes of Health, Bethesda, MD.

Fox N.F., Chan J.K., Tharner M, et al. (1997). Medical expenditures for the treatment of osteoporosis fractures in the United States in 1995: Report from the National Osteoporosis Foundation. *Journal of Bone and Mineral Research, 12,* 24-35.

Gallagher J.C., Rapuri P.B., Haynatzki G., Detter J.R. (2002). Effect of discontinuation of estrogen calcitriol, and the combination of both on bone density and bone markers. *Journal of Clinical Endocrinology & Metabolism, 87,* 4914-4923.

Holt, Stephen. M.D. (2002). The Antiporosis Plan: A Wellness Guide. Wellness Publishing. Newark, NJ.

Kanis J.A., for the WHO study group. (1994). Assessment of fracture risk and its application to screening for postmenopausal osteoporosis: synopsis of a WHO report. *Osteoporosis International,* 4,368-361.

Leonetti H., M.D., Longo S., M.D., Anasti J., M.D. (1999). Transdermal Progesterone Cream for Vasomotor Symptoms and Postmenopausal Bone Loss. *Obstetrics and Gynecology*, January, 94 (2), 225-228.

Marshall D., Johnell Q., Wedel H. (1996). Meta-analysis of how well measures of bone mineral density predict occurrence of osteoporotic fractures. *British Medical Journal, 372*, 1254-1259.

Prestwood K.M., Kenny A.M., Kleppinger A., Kulldorff M. (2003). Ultralow-Dose Micronized 17-Estradiol and Bone Density and Bone Metabolism in Older Women: A Randomized Controlled Trial.*The Journal of the American Medical Association, 290*,1042-1048.

Siris E.S., Miller P.D., Barrett-Connor E., et al. (2001). Identification and fracture outcomes of undiagnosed low bone mineral density in postmenopausal women: results from the National Osteoporosis Risk Assessment. *The Journal of the American Medical Association, 286*, 2815-2822.

Writing Group for the Women's Health Initiative. (2002). Risks and benefits of estrogen plus progestin in health menopausal women. *The Journal of the American Medical Association, 288*, 321-333.

Chapter 8

Alexander J.L.M.D., F.A.B.P.N., F.R.C.P.C., Kotz, K. Ph.D., M.P.H., Dennerstein L., A.O., M.B.B.S., Ph.D., D.P.M., F.R.A.N.Z.C.P., Davis S.R., M.B., B.S, F.R.A.C.P., Ph.D., (2003). The Systemic Nature of Sexual Functioning in the Postmenopausal Woman: Crossroads of Psychiatry and Gynecology. *Primary Psychiatry 10* (12), 53-37.

Bachmann G.A. (1985). Correlates of Sexual Desire in Postmenopausal Women. *Maturitas, 7*(3), 211.

Cohen I., Speroff L., (1981). Premature Ovarian Failure: Update. *Obstetrics and Gynecologic Survey, 47* (3).

Coulam C.B., Adamson S.C., Annegers J.F. (1986). Incidence of Premature Ovarian Failure. *American Journal of Obstertics and Gynecology, 67* (4.)

Doyle L.L. et al., (1971). Human Luteal Function Following Hysterectomy as Assessed by Plasma Progestin. *American Journal of Obstetrics and Gynecology, 110.*

Hargrove J., et al., (1989). Menopausal Hormone Replacement Therapy with Continuous Daily Oral Micronized Estradiol and Progesterone. *Obstetrics and Gynecology, 73* (4), 606-612.

Hung T.T. et al., (1989). Artificially Induced Menstrual Cycle with Natural Estradiol and Progesterone. *Fertility and Sterility, 51*(6).

Longscope C., Jaffe W., Griffing G., (1981). Production Rates of Androgens and Oestrogens in Post-Menopausal Women. *Maturitas, 3,* 215-223

Siddle N., Sarrel P., Whitehead M. (1987). The Effect of Hysterectomy on the Age of Ovarian Failure: Identification of a Subgroup of Women with Premature Loss of Ovarian Function and Literature Review. *Fertility and Sterility, 47* (1).

Speroff L., M.D. (2003). Efficacy and Tolerability of a Novel Estradiol Baginal Ring for Relief of Menopausal Symptoms. *The American College of Obstetricians and Gynecologists, 102*(4), 823.

Young D. (1993). Common Misconceptions About Sex and Depression During Menopause: A Historical Perspective. *Female Patient 17,* 25-28.

Zussman L et al., (1981). Sexual Response After Hysterectomy-Oophorectomy: Recent Studies and Reconsideration of

Psychogenesis. *American Journal of Obstetrics and Gynecology, 140* (7), 725-729.

Chapter 9

Cutter C.B., M.D. (2004). Androgen Deficiency in Women: Understanding the Science, Controversy and Art of Treating our Patients – Part 1. *International Journal of Pharmaceutical Compounding, 8*(1),16.

Graham JD, Clarke CL. Physiological action of pro-gesterone in target tissues. *Endocrine Reviews, 18*, 502-519.

Wilsom, James l. (2001). *Adrenal Fatigue.* Smart Publications. Petaluma, CA

Wright JV. (1999). Comparative measurements of serum estriol, estradiol, and E1 in non-pregnant, premenopausal women; A preliminary investigation. *Alternative Medicine Review, 4*, 266-270.

Schechter D. (1999). Estrogen, progesterone, and mood. *Journal of Gender Specific Medicine, 2*, 29-36.

Chapter 10

Bergkvist L., Adami H.O., Persson L. et al., (1989). The Risk of Breast Cancer After Estrogen and Estrogen-Progestin Replacement. *New England Journal of Medicine, 321*, 293-297.

Colditz G.A. et al., Prospective Study of Estrogen Replacement Therapy and Risk of Breast Cancer in Postmenopausal Women. *The Journal of the American Medical Association, 264*,2648-2652.

Hargrove JT, Maxson WS, Wentz C, et al. (1989). Menopausal hormone replace-ment therapy with continuous daily oral micronized estradiol and proges-terone. *Obstetrics & Gynecology, 73*, 606-612.

Lemon H. et al., (1966). Reduced Estriol Excretion in Patients with Breast Cancer Prior to Endocrine Therapy. *The Journal of the American Medical Association, 196*, 1128-1136.

Lemon H.M. (1975). Estriol Prevention of Mammary Carcinoma Induced by 7, 12-Dimethylbenzanthracene and Procarbazine. *Cancer Research*, 35, 1341-1353.

Lemon H. (1980). Pathophysiologie Considerations in the Treatment of Menopausal Patients with Oestrogens; The Prevention of Mammary Carcinoma. *Acta Endocrinology*, 17-27.

Gambrell, Jr. R.D. (1992). Complications of Estrogen Replacement Therapy. In Swartz D.P. ed., *Hormone Replacement Therapy* (Baltimore, MD: Williams and Wilkins, 1992), Chapter 9.

Shi-Zhong B, De-Ling Y, Xiu-Hai R, et al. (1997). Progesterone induces apoptosis and up-regulation of p53 expression in human ovarian carcinoma cell lines. *Cancer, 79*, 10.

Siller-Arenas et al., (1990). Menopausal Hormone Replacement Therapy and Breast Cancer: A Meta-Analysis. *Obstetrics and Gynecology, 79* (2).

Yu S, Lee M, Shin S, et al. (2001). Apoptosis induced by progesterone in human ovarian cancer cell line SNU-840. *Journal of Cellular Biochemistry, 82,* 445-451.

Wetiz H.H., Beebe D.R., Muller E. (Rp. 1984). Effect of Estrogens on DMBA-Induced Breast Tumors. *Journal of Steriod Biochemistry, 20,* 1067-1075.

Chapter 11

Aldercreutz H. et al., Dietary Phyto-oestrogens and the Menopause in Japan. *Lancet 339,* 1233.

Adlercreutz H., et al. (1982). Excretion of the Lignans Enterolactone and Enterodiol and of Equol in Omnivorous and Vegetarian Postmenopausal Women and in Women With Breast Cancer. *Lancet, 2* (8311), 1295-1299.

Campagnoli C., et al. (1999). HRT and Breast Cancer Risk: A Clue for Interpreting the Available Data. *Maturitas, 33,* 185-190.

Chen C. C., et al. (1995). Adverse Life Events and Breast Cancer: Case-Control Study. *British Medical Journal, 311,* 1527-1530.

Clemetson C.A.B., DeCarol S.J., Burney G.A., Patel T.J., Kozhiashvili N., et al., (1978). Estrogens in Food: The Almond Mystery. *International Journal of Gynecology and Obstetrics, 15,* 515-521.

Collaborative Group on Hormonal Factors in Breast Cancer (1997). Breast Cancer and Hormone Replacement Therapy: Collaborative Reanalysis of Data from 51 Epidemiological Studies of 52,705 Women with Breast Cancer and 108,411 Without Breast Cancer. *Lancet, 350,* 1047-1059.

Elakovich S.O., Hampton J., (1984). Analysis of Couvaestrol, A Phytoestrogen, in Alpha Tablets Sold for Human Consumption. *Journal of Agricultural Food Chemistry 32,* 173-175.

Goldin B.R., Adlercreutz H., et al (1982). Estrogen Excretion Patterns and Plasma Levels in Vegetarian and Omnivorous Women. *New England Medical Journal, 307,* 1542-1547.

Kerlikowske K., et al. (1993). Positive Predictive Value of Screening Mammography By Age and Family History of Breast Cancer. *The Journal of the American Medical Association, 270* (2), 444.

LaVecchia C., Negri E., Franceschi S., et al. (1995). Hormone Replacement Therapy and Breast Cancer Risk: A Cooperative Italian Study. *British J. Cancer, 72,* 244-248.

Lee W., Harder J., Yoshizumi M., et al (1997). Progesterone Inhibits Arterial Smooth Muscle Cell Proliferation. *Natural Medicine, 3,* 1005-1008.

Leonetti H., Longo S., Anasti J. (2003). Topical Progesterone Cream has an Antiproliferative Effect on Estrogen-Stimulated Endometrium. *Obstetrics & Gynecology,* 79, 221-222.

Levy S., et al. (1987). Correlation of Stress Factors with Sustained Depression of Natural Killer Cell Activity and Predicted Prognosis in Patients With Breast Cancer. *Journal of Clinical Oncology, 5,* 348-353.

Lundstrom E., Wilczek B., von Palffy Z., et al. (2001). Mammographic Breast Density During Hormone Replacement Therapy: Effects of Continuous Combination, Unopposed Transdermal and Low-Potency Estrogen Regimens. *Climacteric 4,* 42-48.

Phillips K.A. (1999). Putting the Risk of Breast Cancer in Perspective. *New England Medical Journal, 340 (2),* 141-144.

Reed M., Purohit A. (1997). Breast Cancer and the Role of Cytokines in Regulating Estrogen Synthesis: an Emerging Hypothesis. *Endocrine Reviews, 18,* 701-715.

Toikkanene S., et al. (1991). Factors Predicting Late Mortality from Breast Cancer. *European Journal of Cancer, 27* (5), 586-591.

Weisberg T. (1996). Genetic Testing for Breast Cancer. *Maine Cancer Perspectives, 2 (4),* 3.

Willet W.C., et al. (1987). Moderate Alcohol Consumption and the Risk of Breast Cancer. *New England Medical Journal, 316,* 1174-1180.

Chapter 12

(2001). Testosterone Therapy: Spotlight On The Older Man At Last. *Health & Medicine Week.*

(2002). Hormone replacement therapy safe for most men with andropause. (In The Public Eye). *Urology Times, 30*(10), 16.

(2003). Male Menopause linked to higher risk of heart disease. *Heart Disease Weekly, 2.*

(2003). On Call – Hormone replacement therapy for men. (Letter to the Editor). *Harvard Men's Health Watch, 7* (6).

(2003). Sexual dysfunction and andropause lead strong growth in men's segment. *Drug Week,* 279

(2004). Hormone therapy leads to high rates of osteoporosis in men. *Drug Week,* 411.

Channer, K.S., & Jones, T.H., (2003). Cardiovascular effects of testosterone: implications of the 'male menopause'? (Editorial) *Heart,* 89(2),121-123.

CMP Information Ltd. (2004). Is there a male menopause and should we treat it? *Pulse,* 62.

Cutler, B. (1993). Marketing to menopausal men *American Demographics* 15(3), 49

Gould D.C., Petty R., & Jacobs H.S. (2000). The male menopause-does it exist? *British Medical Journal,* V320(7238), 858.

Groopman, J. (2002). Hormones for Men. *The New Yorker.*

Jenkins, T. (1995). Male menopause: myth or monster? *Vibrant Life,*11(6), 12-15.

Meagher, J. (2003). Is male menopause just a myth? *Europe Intelligence Wire.*

Naish, J. (2003). HRT for men? I don't believe it: is the male menopause fact or fiction? As John Naish reports, there is increasing controversy about treating men of certain age with testosterone. *Nursing Standard,* 17(37), 202

Quallich, A.S. (2003). Andropause. *Urologic Nursing,* 23(4), 301-302.

Sinclair J.F., Niederberger C.S. & Meacham R.B. (2003). Diagnosing androgen deficiency in the aging male. *Contemporary Urology,* 15(4), 70-75.

Ulrich, M. (2001). Men who maunder about their fading virility should learn to grow old gracefully. *The Report Newsmagazine.*

Index

ABOUT THE AUTHORS

C. W. (Randy) Randolph, Jr., M. D.

Dr. Randolph is internationally recognized for his natural medicine approach to women's health concerns. As a trained pharmacist and Board Certified practicing physician, Dr. Randolph has treated thousands of women suffering from the symptoms of hormone imbalance. For more than a decade, Dr. Randolph has built a sound foundation of clinical evidence to support the safety and efficacy of treating patients with human-identical hormones (e.g. estrogens, progesterone, testosterone) versus synthetic hormone replacement therapies (HRT).

Dr. Randolph was first trained as a pharmacist and graduated from Auburn University's School of Pharmacy. He then received his medical doctoral education at Louisiana State University's School of Medicine in New Orleans, Louisiana. In concert with his belief in the efficacy of natural medicine, Dr. Randolph has sought out continuing medical educational forums emphasizing the value of more holistic and natural approaches to patient care and treatment. In 2000, he completed an intensive training on integrated medicine at Columbia University Medical School.

In addition to his multi-faceted clinical expertise and his professional credibility, Dr. Randolph evidences great success as an entrepreneur and business leader within the medical community. In 2003, he founded The Natural Hormone Institute of America in order to formalize a business entity committed to the ongoing research and development of human-identical hormone therapies. In addition, in early 2004 Dr. Randolph determined to work with Genie James and Rick Buchsbaum to co-found a company - LIVESSE, LLC - that could respond to the promptings and requests of many of his physician peers who were increasingly contacting him with an interest in learning more about his practice model and, ultimately, replicating his clinical and business success. Today, LIVESSE brings to physicians a franchising opportunity for adding natural/complementary medicine and human-identical hormone products into a medical practice.

As a result of his commitment to a more caring and informed approach to treating women's health concerns, Dr. Randolph is celebrated as a physician champion of natural medicine and women's health, as well as a pioneer in the realms of personalized medicine and natural hormone therapies. By founding The Natural Hormone Institute of America and LIVESSE, LLC, Dr. Randolph continues to expand his commitment to a mission to improve the traditional healthcare delivery system by championing patient advocacy, physician training and, most specifically, human-identical hormone therapies.

Dr. Randolph was born and raised in Apalachicola, a small town in the panhandle of Florida. He feels that his heightened awareness as to the importance of listening and caring is most probably derived from having been nurtured in a community where everyone was known and everyone's concerns mattered. As a physician of natural medicine, Dr. Randolph believes that it has been the love of his family that has provided him with the stamina and courage to forge into realms of medicine that were previously somewhat controversial. As a healer, Dr. Randolph humbly acknowledges that his talents are derived from a Higher Power and it is his privilege to serve others with his work.

Genie James, M.M.Sc.
Ms. James has over 20 years of experience developing and executing business development and revenue growth initiatives

for health systems and physician groups. For more than 10 out of the last 15 years, Ms. James has run her own consulting business focusing on strategic business development and new program/product launch while also emphasizing the critical importance of personalized medicine and relationship-centered care. Through hands-on experience, Ms. James has developed a unique expertise specific to women's health initiatives and complementary/integrated healthcare initiatives.

From 2000 to 2002, Ms. James served as Vice President of Sales, Marketing and Managed Care for American HomePatient. Prior to that, Ms. James served as Executive Vice President of Managed Care and Marketing for PrincipalCare, Inc., a women's health physician practice management firm. Ms. James has a Masters of Medical Science (M.M.Sc.) from Emory University. She is also the author of two books: *Making Managed Care Work* and *Winning In The Women's HealthCare Marketplace*.